# *Healing* *Cancer*
## with the
## Power of Your Mind

Published by Rudy Kachmann, M.D. Kachmann Media, LLC
www.KachmannMindBody.com

Library of Congress Control Number: TO COME
ISBN-10: 1463745265
EAN-13: 9781463745264
Gary Ritter, Editor
Printed in the United States of America

# Healing Cancer
## with the
# Power of Your Mind

## Love - Hope - Faith

Dr. Rudy Kachmann,
Neurosurgeon

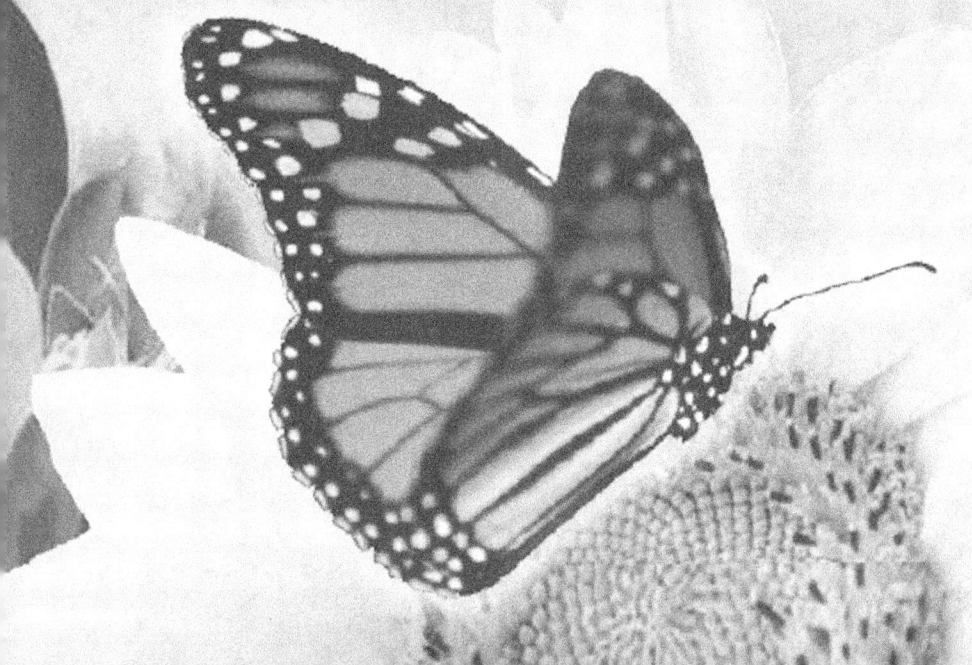

# Contents

# Preface

The incidence of cancer is common today. Oncology, radiation, and medicine are not hard to find for most patients. Many cannot afford the latest chemotherapy programs or experimental drugs to save their lives. Many times the insurance companies don't want to pay for them, as they can cost 20 to 100 thousand dollars a year. What is not easy to find—and, as a matter of fact, sometimes impossible to find—is teaching the patients how to mobilize their self-healing abilities and bring these to the aid of cancer treatment. This book will review the science behind the powers of the mind in the healing process. The mind-cancer connection indeed has great power, and I will explain the science of it and encourage you to participate in the process and take advantage of this modality of healing. It goes back to the days of Hippocrates and it's playing a larger part in treatments year after year. Many cancer specialists have little knowledge in this field and have admitted that to me.

Our thoughts do affect our body chemistry, hormones, neurotransmitters, and neuropeptides that connect the mind to the body and the body to the mind. Every one of our thoughts affects seventy trillion body cells. It has been scientifically proven that the immune system—your army, navy, and air force—is greatly affected by this thought process. Happiness, hopefulness, hopelessness, and depression greatly affect your immunity, in a good or bad way depending on your thought process.

This book is written for patients and providers. The idea is to promote a holistic approach, to connect the physiology, anatomy, pathology, psychology, and spiritual aspect of the illness. The whole being: mind-body, body-mind.

My previous book, *Welcome to Your Mind Body*, explains the science of mind-body medicine. I clearly recommend that you participate in your chemo and radiation treatments, but in addition consider the power of your mind and its ability to heal the body.

# Hopefulness, Love, and Healing

We finally have started to connect the brain back with the body. Years ago, to suggest that the mind affects your health would cause disbelief, although it has been known since the time of Aristotle in 400 BC. All of a sudden, love, hopefulness, music, and exercise are being promoted as healing modalities.

Prophets, witch doctors, and holistic healers have handed down healing and survival techniques to us for thousands of years. The placebo effect has been known for thousands of years; "I believe, and I get better." Snake oil and leeches even worked at times. Thousands of articles have been published on the placebo effect. An awareness of one's mortality can lead one to wake up and live an authentic, meaningful life. This can have a great effect on healing from cancer or any other mind-body illness.

The issue is about living a better, longer, and more purposeful life.

The mind and body are one; one integrated system. How we eat, think, exercise, and feel are related to our health. Physicians need to have this knowledge, which many do not, to teach the mind-body connection. The famous book by Dr. Candace Pert, *Molecules of Emotion*, is a good source of information about that. My book *Welcome to Your Mind Body* discusses in great detail the science of the mind-body connection, and also what I call mind-body illnesses. My most grateful patients are the ones I teach the mind-body connection to. Seventy-five percent of the patients seeing a doctor just need good coaching. Physicians need to be technicians, knowing how to prescribe, but also following through with the mind-body connection. They also need to incorporate philosophy and spirituality into their treatment. When one's existence is threatened there are more issues and questions to confront than just medication and surgery. We need a team approach—patient, health-care provider, family, and spirituality. The doctor and patient need to invest in each other.

We lose our authentic life when we give in to the demands of others, or we become something other than what we want to be in order to get their love or simply just to be cared for. When we awaken to our own mortality, and if we plan to get well, we refuse to live the life that is killing us and start living in being our own true self. On a practical level it may mean changing occupations, moving, changing the way we eat or exercise, or developing new relationships and ending old relationships, bringing meaning and a new attitude to life. If you don't bring forth what is within you, what you have may destroy you. If you bring forth what is within you, what you bring forth will heal you.

The ancients were healers of body and mind, a very powerful tool, promoting hopefulness and spirituality. Survivors take time to be still and listen. It can be medicine, surgery, imaging, relaxation, art, or music, but it all amounts to finding time to be still and listen to the voice within you. Sir William Osler, the great doctor from Canada and medical historian, said, "It is more important to know what's going on in the patient's mind than in his lungs." He was working in a TB sanatorium at the beginning of the last century. Obviously, he was talking about the effects of the mind on a person's immunity. Hippocrates said he would rather know what sort of person has a disease than what sort of disease that person has. Louis Pasteur and Claude Bernard argued all their lives about whether the most important factor in disease was "the soil" or germ in the human body. Was it the mind or the bacteria? On his deathbed Pasteur, the father of the germ theory of illness, admitted to Bernard that he was right, declaring, "It is the soil."

Most doctors seldom consider or connect the patient's attitude, shape of his life, or the quality or quantity of it to the patient's illness. Patients vary in their response. We offer a choice between operation and a change in lifestyle. About 80 percent say, "Operate." That probably is still true today. People want a procedure, and only about 20 percent are willing to participate actively in the healing process. I've noticed that in the field of back pain and surgery they don't have to do the work and it's a lot easier than weight loss and exercise. When I have promoted a wellness approach, I have received some nasty letters back, and a number of times patients complained that I did not address the basic problem. They wanted a quick fix. That's why we have so much unnecessary surgery on the back today, with many poor results.

The ability to love is not limited by the body's illness, according to Dr. Bernie S. Siegel. I recommend his book *Love, Medicine and Miracles* highly; I am quoting from it. Scientific research and Dr. Siegel's day-to-day experience convinced him that the state of mind changes the state of the body, working through the central nervous system, the endocrine system, and the immune system. Peace of mind sends the body a "live" message, while depression, fear, and conflict give it a "die" message. Even science can't explain the unexpected "miracle cure." The fundamental problem is that most patients face an inability to love themselves. Miracles don't come from the cold intellect. We must give the patient the option to participate in recovery from cancer or any other type of illness. Death is not the issue, life is. Death is not a failure. Dr. Norman Vincent Peale, in his many famous books on positive thinking, says we must remove the word *impossible* from our vocabulary; "you can if you think you can." We need to switch to the creative mode, away from the destructive mode, according to Dr. Sigmund Freud. Anyone who does not believe in miracles is not a realist.

In 1978, Dr. Carl Simonton and his wife published a famous study of cancer patients. They use imaging techniques against cancer, mind-body techniques.

The report was on total cancer patients who had only about a year to live, 159 of them. Ninety percent got rid of the cancer completely, the disease was regressed in another 20 percent, and they lived twice as long as the non-treated patients. The Simontons taught the patients how to meditate and visualize; subjects we will discuss later in the book.

One problem with cancer statistics is that the miracle cures are not reported. If we could only scientifically prove how one of those got better, it would be a revolution in cancer treatment. Dr. Bernie Siegel found that 15 to 20 percent of patients actually want to die, and they do. Dr. Siegel found that 60 to 70 percent of patients just do what the doctor wants them to do and don't participate in their treatment. Operate equals "I don't have to do anything; I don't have to eat right, I don't have to exercise, and I don't need to learn mind-body techniques." As I already mentioned, I found the same thing in treating back pain. They want the doctor to do the work. They take the pills and have the surgery done, but they don't strike out for themselves. Given a choice, they would rather be operated on. The aggressive, positive thinker—"I'm not going to die"—is much more likely to get well. It has been found that aggressive patients have more killer T cells—our army, navy, and air force that defend our body. Patients with a fighting spirit get better at a rate of 75 percent, versus 22 percent for the stoic, nonparticipating patient. A question I commonly ask patients is if they want to live to be one hundred and be of sound mind and sound body. I tell them I can teach them how to do it, and if they participate many get better, live longer, and the spontaneous cure rate goes up. Health-care providers, especially oncologists, rarely have a positive attitude, and that is a problem. If you are told, "You have only six months to live," that is exactly what will happen—and you should run from that doctor! Dr. Siegel feels, and I agree, that doctors should be required to attend holistic healing seminars, in which people cured of diseases get to talk. Wouldn't it be a great medical meeting, like one Dr. Ben Siegel went to, with 50 percent patients and 50 percent health-care providers? We would all learn something from that.

# The Will to Live

We need to connect the mind to the body. How we think has a great effect on our health. In her famous book *Molecules of Emotion*, Candace Pert clearly explains the science behind the mind-body connection. Our brains speak to our body through hormones, neurotransmitters, and neuropeptides—especially to our immune system, the army, navy, and air force defending us from cancer and foreign invaders. All of us develop a few cancer cells every day, and if immunity is intact we eliminate or repair those cells. Interestingly enough, our white cells, our immunity, also make neuropeptides, about 350, that in turn speak to our body and brain—the mind-body, body-mind. When we have cancer, clearly our immunity is critical to our survival. How we think and act can have a great effect on the outcome. The will to live is critical to our survival. Many die when told the diagnosis of cancer. What they don't understand is that today, with our present treatments, at least 50 percent of patients are cured, and another 25 percent live many years. You can see that actually there is great hope, and that participation of the patient is critical. Some people literally will themselves to death. I have seen it a number of times. Then again, I've had patients who said, "I'm not going to die," and a number of those had a spontaneous cure and many lived a lot longer than expected. That has been the experience of many well-known physicians and is well described in their books, which I will refer to extensively. We are finally moving toward the recognition that in an illness of any kind, from the common cold to cancer, emotional stress plays a huge part. We have a powerful doctor within us that can keep us alive. Miracles of healing have been done by faith, positive thinking, and a mind-body connection produced by hopefulness. Many of those cases cannot be explained by medical science unless we include the power of the human mind.

Anxiety is one of the signs that the "will to live" is under attack. Depression goes a step further; it indicates a partial surrender to death.

Anxiety shows in the mind that all life is threatened. A remote possibility, to the anxious mind, becomes a possibility. Anxiety disrupts our body's normal functioning. A skin rash can be due to a change in body chemistry. Anxiety is the whisper of danger from the unconscious; whether it is real or imagined makes no difference. The threat of cancer to health is real and depression is a partial surrender to death.

"A tranquil mind is a well-ordered mind," and supports the will to live. You can see how important the mind is in treating cancer. A person in conflict is like a country in a state of civil war. A schizophrenic has given up reality to survive; that is his or her expression of the will to live. Psychotics have great health, a dream world with no stress. Sigmund Freud said we have two instincts, the destructive instinct and the creative instinct. Man turns his creative and destructive impulse upon himself. Illness is the unconscious, temporary surrender of the will to live.

Repeated illness is a form of slow suicide. Why does one survive and another die? The will to live makes a great difference because the neurochemicals of the brain affect immunity. There is an increased rate of cancer in spouses within a year if their mate dies. For some, life without love has no value. There are many stories in medical literature and newspapers that reflect this. Christopher Reeve died and his wife, with no history of smoking, died of lung cancer within the year. There are many stories like that. The emotion of love may determine the vitality of the will to live or the wish to die. Emotional stress and physical stress lead to disease. Love is as healing and as potent as drugs. Man dies when he wants to die. Conscious or unconscious, we make our own choice. Fear of death is universal. "Come, Sweet Death" is a famous song by Bach. We may fear pain when actually, with today's medicines, cancer patients have very little pain.

What we really fear is that life will end before we are ready, that we'll die before we've had a chance to make our mark. We die only when we are ready to die. When we want to live, we may die because unconsciously we want to die, although we may convince ourselves and others that we have things to live for.

If we truly wish to live, and we have incentives to live, we have something; no matter how sick we are, we do not die. The incentives must be ones which we believe in, inwardly and utterly. We must meet our own uncompromising reasoning, or knowledge, of what is worth living for. You need a purpose, especially if the diagnosis is cancer, or any other life-threatening and debilitating illnesses.

There have been many unexpected miracles of healing without clear explanation. The will to live and its effect on you through your immunity may be the answer.

Deep within every living thing exists the will to live. The purpose is to preserve it; it is wired in nature. Your immunity has great power. It works for you every day. It's the keystone of every organic existence. So strong is it for man and animal alike that both will fight desperately to keep life going, no matter how wretched life may be. The biological will to live may not be enough to support us through the complexities of life in a civilized world. We need moral and emotional force to make the struggle enduring.

Last year I had a young patient with a tennis-ball-sized tumor in his neck. He was a smoker. I asked him to visualize a Pac-Man coming in and eating up the tumor. He was to meet me nine months later on my dock at the lake, where we normally did some fishing, for lunch. I set the date and time, and nine months later he arrived with four big bass on a stringer. We cleaned and ate them. This type of story is what Dr. Carl Simonton speaks about in his books. Every extraordinary man has a mission which he is called upon to fulfill. Goethe died when his mission, *Faust*, was done. Every human being aspires to some achievement; it may be clear or clouded in his or her unconscious mind.

We all have our own goals; we all evaluate ourselves and our subconscious mind. We play out our own destiny and will have our own unique way of dealing with it. Some individuals rebel against what's happening and others get to work. Whether the individual accepts life with these things or rejects it, will determine the course of it.

How is power passed from the creative to the destructive drive? Why does the will to live weaken before the wish to die? When reason and emotion are locked in battle, emotion eventually wins. Can we guard ourselves against the shift of power from the life-preserving force? Can we surrender the will to live? The best way to prolong life is not to shorten it. The first line of defense is our own emotional life. If we are emotionally sound, we will be physically sound. Body and mind are one. When we truly want to be well, to live long and in health, we have the power to do it. "Live for your own sake, we need you." We need to guard our emotions and our physical health. Many retire and die quickly. No one needs to fear death, because we die only when we're ready. We need a reason to live; we need to work on living, not dying. The knowledge that the body cannot be healed without the mind goes back to Socrates in 500 BC. The destructive drive is an ever-ready force lurking in the unconscious mind. When we cease to release our creative energies, when we are caught in emotional conflict, then the mind's emotional structure can become an actual threat to our health. The destructive drive is forever lurking—"I give up, I don't want to live"—it's the unconscious mind at work. When we fail to release our creative energies, we are blocked; we're caught in the toils of emotional conflict, and the destructive impulse can activate and threaten our health. If we recognize the destructive impulse and act to remove it, we can prevent illness.

The illness of cancer does not come out of the blue. Cancer can be a response to stress. The steroids secreted by stress destroy our immunity. Years ago, when I had no partners in the practice of neurosurgery and worked day and night, I would frequently get a cold on Saturday and by Sunday I would be well. My immunity had been compromised by stress. When my first partner arrived, he developed the same problem because he was not used to working that hard. When the third partner arrived we were all well. Fear without cause, fatigue, and multiple small illnesses—all can be warning signs that our immunity is being compromised. Guilt can be stressful. Guilt implies punishment, and the superego is relentless and may destroy you. After a divorce, breakdowns, cancer, or death are common. A lost job can do the same. People who are at odds with themselves have a narrow margin of safety. Under stress, the unconscious gives warning signs to be healed by those who wish to live in health. Life confronts everyone with stressful situations and stress causes wear and tear on the body. Whether the stress is external or internal, the wear and tear is the same. Cancer may be the result. We may select our illness; we may subconsciously choose the time of illness, the course, and its gravity. We don't reason ourselves into illness; decisions are made by the unconscious mind. We choose the time of illness. "I'm not going to die," a patient of mine said, and he lived ten years with a horrible cancer. I helped him with positive thinking. I gave him the books of Dr. Norman Vincent Peale to read. Long-term stress can lead to cancer. It destroys immunity and your eicosanoids—your Intel chips. We can escape into illness. Sometimes we use illness to develop a new perspective. Sometimes it can even be lifesaving. Illness can be shock therapy, convalescing can be a time for taking stock. It may improve our immunity and cure the problem. It may give us time to make decisions and lay out a new course. Some have a death wish and want to escape the world. Illness now fulfills a need, separating us from the problem. Perhaps we feel unable to solve the problem; perhaps we are unable to face it. Illness may be an unconscious device to change a situation and change people's attitude toward us. Cancer may be a way of putting us in a different situation. But its duration into illness, however long or short, for whatever reason, is costly to ourselves and to those close to us.

## The Mind and Immunity

We live longer, maybe double our life span and even increase the spontaneous cure rate, by mobilizing our compromised immune system and following a purpose in living. Dr. Lawrence LeShan, in his famous and great book *Cancer As a Turning Point*, taught his patients to mobilize the self-healing mechanisms and bring the process to the aid of standard medical treatment. He found that, in treating thousands of patients, if he could get one to develop a purpose in his or her life, and develop some meaning for his or her living, that many times he could turn the whole cancer case around. People started living longer and more spontaneous cures occurred. As a psychotherapist, he felt he needed to change his approach to cancer. He needed to ask his patients, "What is right with you? What is the most natural way for you to live and train the creative, not the destructive, path? What kind of life and lifestyle make you glad to get up in the morning, glad to go to bed at night, and give you maximum zest and enthusiasm for living? What kind of life would you be living if your purpose or actual ambition could be accomplished?" He would ask his cancer patients, "If your fairy godmother is coming to earth in five minutes, and is willing to grant you a wish for any new way of living or a new career, what would interest you? What might put zest in your life, give you something to look forward to, something that you could work for, a reason for living?" He gave patients only a short period of time so the real story might come out. Then, if possible, he would encourage the patients to work toward that goal.

Therapy is useful for mobilizing cancer patients' immune systems and aims to discovering that answer, in understanding what has sparked a person's perception of himself or what the driving force in his or her lifestyle is. Very often, the patient will respond with, "I don't know" when asked what changes in life he or she might be interested in. The goal then becomes having to accept what the most important quest at this stage of his or her life is. Mere acceptance of the quest and a commitment to finding out the answer quickly had a positive effect on a patient's immune system and he or she improved. Patients responded better and more effectively to their medical protocol when they had an emotional acceptance and made a commitment to the treating process. The therapist must have a clear understanding of the patient's psychology and must communicate repeatedly that patient's commitment to the future. The pathology of the cancer, the actual tumor, can be put in a more hopeful light, and still be realistic in most cases. "You have only six months to live" is just not going to do it. None of us can predict everything 100 percent, and there are always exceptions. Statements like "Ten percent of the people actually do quite well in some very serious cases" will in fact give a lot of patients some hope and a reason to develop a purpose to their life. The therapeutic process has a different flavor and will have different results. Hopefulness has great power and mobilizes the immune system. The mind can mobilize neuropeptides, hormones, and neurotransmitters that affect our whole body and immune system. This type of therapy depends on real "encounters"; authentic contact between the therapist and client. Certainly, many patients can do this without a therapist. Many can cross the mountain alone; we don't all need a guide.

We can ask the patient, "How would you design a way of life for you that you will enjoy for a long time? One in which you will relate, create, give, and take the right way for you?" I always say this particular phrasing should be used for people with particularly intellectual backgrounds. However, the general approach is the idea. Encourage the patient to set out to make sure there is some enjoyment in his or her life. For many, a new career is not possible, but there are lots of additional things we can do besides work that would make every day more meaningful for us. As you look at your life, what were the best moments? What were those moments that you remember as the peaks? After exploring these, the therapist goes on to help the patient find what the patient said in comments and in what themes of this particular individual's life history they celebrated and then expanded. Then the explanation goes on—how a life could be set up, what it could be like—so that there would be as many of these moments as possible. From this, one continues to build an understanding of the kind of life that would be the most fulfilling. Find out what's right with you! Negativity could be a natural way of being, but it's ugly and repellent, and we must get rid of it. Only creativity will cause us to survive; destructive thinking has no value. When people with cancer were presented with this concept and set goals, then negative reactions frequently fell into one or more of these classes. I found my own music, but it was so discordant, I wouldn't like it and no one else would, either. My own natural way of being was ugly and repellent, and I learned a long time ago not to express it if I wanted to have any relationships and be able to live with myself. If I found my own song and tried to sing it, I would find there was no place in the world for anyone like me. I couldn't support myself if I was living the song that is right for me. My own song would have such contradictions built into it that it would be impossible. The above reasons certainly are quite understandable. Many of us cannot change the circumstances of our lives because of obligations and financial restrictions. That doesn't mean that we can't change our way of thinking. Then again, the experience of Dr. Lawrence LeShan was that he never saw a single person who, upon finding his or her own song and style, still felt the same. He said he never encountered an exception to that. You need to find your music; it will change your outcome. We all have a unique song to sing, completely individual music with its own beat which, when it is found, generally has three characteristics. It was joyful for the person, socially positive, and improved his or her human relationships. Give a man a mission and just working toward it can be lifesaving. All people have a natural way of being, relating, and creating. When they find it, they use themselves in the way that is most fulfilling. It is also my experience that when patients become committed to finding and then living this new way, their body's defenses increase their functioning, and they frequently begin to respond much more positively to whatever medical treatment they were on.

I like to encourage all people with cancer to seek a lifestyle that is uniquely theirs. We need to look to you as an individual, since we're all different, and treat you in a holistic manner. Each relationship is unique. You need to develop an album of sketches of the landscape, a mind map. You can draw it and help illuminate the terrain. Every person's psychology is different and that must be kept in mind. You must take some control over your own life, searching for a lifestyle especially suited for you, and when you find it, actively work toward living this life. What would fulfill you? What style of being, relating, and creating would bring you to a life of zest? This is the life, live in the search for it. It will mobilize the immune system against cancer more than anything else we know today. I know it works. Your future is based on your genetic inheritance, your life experience, and your reaction to it. Doing the same thing over and over again and expecting it to turn out differently may not work for you. You may need to think outside the box. Common sense is not always the best process.

# The Problem of Despair or Hopelessness

Some people believe, in a deep and profound orientation, that no matter what they do they cannot bring any real meaning, zest, or enthusiasm to their life. The word *cancer* itself can put patients straight into depression. They may die quickly, overcome by a state of futility, hopelessness, and depression. Psychologists have found that despair is the basic life orientation that emerges in many cancer patients during treatment. It may go totally unnoticed externally. Its verbalization may come as a surprise to most patients, with the realization that this is the way they actually have felt all along but were not aware of it. Emotional orientation of despair may precede the appearance of cancer by many years. It may actually be the cause and will reduce the patients' immunity. Remember, we all form some cancer cells every day; it's our own immunity that destroys them daily. It has been a persistent feeling for many of the cancer patients all their lives. There were periods when the background music was very loud and times when it was very low, but it always had been there. Once the feeling emerges into consciousness, patients will often be surprised by it for a long time. This can be a difficult time for patients. However, once a realistic orientation has been achieved it can be changed, and the creative process, instead of the destructive process, can begin. Dr. LeShan, in his large study of terminal cancer patients, noticed despair long before the diagnosis of cancer was ever made or confirmed. The problem of their unbearable existence was being solved for them by cancer in a self-destructive psychology. He worked with terminal cancer patients for forty-five years and we should respect his opinion. Nearly all the people he worked with had little hope from medical treatment in the beginning. That was the psychological mind-set of the patients. The basic problem is that the self cannot be expressed to help the healing process. Psychologists say that to get rid of despair one has to reinvent oneself, to bring some meaning and zest to life and in essence become someone else. A different person. For many of us, seeing the truth is very hard and takes time. The solution comes from becoming more and more of who you really are. For too many people, cancer was not seen as something new in their lives, only the latest and final example of their basic hopelessness. The psychological makeup has been part of their existence all along; cancer is just another bump in the road. When I think about it, I've seen it many times.

# The Mind in Cancer Research

Early in his career, Dr. LeShan found that there were increased rates of cancer for widows and widowers that were not related to age, occupation, smoking, or diet. Up to the year 1900, the relationship between cancer and psychology was commonly accepted in medical circles. What happened is quite clear: we had no CT scans, MRIs, or other newfangled tests, and we used to have to talk to people and examine them personally. We really got to know them, so we recognized the psychological factors. Then along came all these fancy tests and now we don't talk to the patient much. If only we'd get know them. So we stopped appreciating the psychological approach to cancer treatment. We are now engineers of the human body. I've said it many times; we should give the new doctors an engineering degree from Purdue instead of a medical degree from Indiana. I see it every day in my practice, in all aspects of medicine. We stopped believing that psychology affects cancer, although the tables are starting to turn again. There is a mind-body connection. We need to ask the patient, "What's going on in your life?" Many of my patients prefer to see the nurse practitioner instead of the family doctor, because he or she will give the patient a hug and say, "What's going on in your life?" The fact is that great emotional loss and hopelessness, occurring well before the first signs of cancer, were seen repeatedly and frequently by the physicians in the 1800s. In 1880, one wrote that cases were so frequent in which depression, anxiety, deferred hope, and disappointment were found in the history of the cancer patients. They hardly doubted that mental depression is common in precancerous conditions. Multiple studies have been done to prove the relationship between psychology and cancer. I have many examples in my practice.

# Develop a Purpose

The highway back to health: "I don't want to die!" Let us not give in to illness; let us make a plan to fight back, because we have the most powerful weapon at our disposal—our mind. We have the army, navy, and marines waiting to fight for us! Our powerful brain! The fight against cancer cannot just be doctors, medicine, surgery, and procedures. Our own way of thinking can be the greatest weapon of all. Let's get to work! Don't let the medical profession do a "nocebo" on you. This negative talk has a voodoo effect. Hear, "I believe there is no hope," and sure enough, you will die when the doctor says you will. I've seen it in my practice time and time again. But I've also seen the effects on the health of a positive thinker. Fear is an obstacle that the doctor must help the patient remove before the patient can be motivated to take action to help himself get well. It's critical to have a loving wellness doctor with a positive personality. The books of Dr. Norman Vincent Peale on positive thinking are great to read. I have read all twenty-one of them; they were given to me by a patient as a gift. Fear can be an emergency. The patient can hide his fear behind a controlled exterior. Fear turns discomfort into pain. Fear builds up over days, weeks, and may increase every month, becoming acute by the time the patient has enough nerve to go to the doctor. Fear must be dealt with promptly. Thinking we harbor a fatal disease when the diagnosis of cancer is made is common. Remember, 50 percent of all cancers are cured, and another 25 percent of patients live for a long time.

There clearly is great hope. People delay treatment because of fear, and delay the healing process because of it. It is a self-destructive act. The doctor must dispel fear with knowledge. In my experience, when I see patients with mind-body illnesses like fibromyalgia, headaches, chronic pain, or even cancer, the best thing I can do is to push knowledge at them. "What is going in your life?" is my opening question. Many times, it's critical. Some people think it's more important to know your patients than the disease that they have. Dr. William Osler said that at the turn of the previous century, and I find it to be true. I provide CDs, DVDs, pamphlets, and books, and give a lot of lectures, including a TV show and radio show, all for patient education. I find that this has been motivating to a significant number of my patients, as well as giving me a great purpose of healing at my young age of thirty-nine—ha!

In order to tap the will to live, the patient has to become an active partner in the process, because this promotes a good patient-doctor relationship.

Often the patient has a feeling of hostility and/or fear of the new specialist, but a loving physician can abate that. A health-care provider must spend a significant amount of time with the patient—no excuses. I'm extremely busy but I seem to find the time! The provider, doctor, nurse, or practitioner must recoup the feeling of caring. "Good afternoon," the issuing of prescriptions, or, "See you later"—these just are not going to do it.

## How to Build the Will to Live

Boredom can be a serious illness. It can be chronic or acute. It's hard to be a positive thinker when you're bored. The creative drive may have surrendered the will to live and we participated in its resignation. Boredom is a total absence of the incentive to go on living. Well-being consists of happiness, joy, and a zest for life. I want to help people. I want to see Johnny graduate from college or get married. Enjoying work and the positive energy that it brings to our lives, including the necessary income, brings rewards, satisfaction of achievement, and recognition. The enjoyment of work and play is a symptom of a flourishing will to live. It is true that our complex industrial civilization often makes it difficult for people to find time to demonstrate their individual creative abilities. Many don't enjoy their work. The solution to the problem is still the same, fight or flight. The creative or destructive impulse of humans is always at play. Either we deal with the situation aggressively and find a solution, or we run. The latter is suicidal. Many grow old before they grow up. The mind is like a muscle; we build it up or we tear it down. The meaning of a man's life is not the length, but the way he conducts it.

## Physician Means Teacher

You cannot teach them anything, you can only help them find it within themselves. A human being is something more than the sum of all medical specialties. The physician must do his duty to teach the patient to become well. I've already mentioned this in many of my CDs, DVDs, and books that I have available for my patients. From proper eating, which is very important in cancer, to stress reduction techniques, exercise techniques, yoga, meditation, positive thinking, and music. Many patients that see a doctor need only a coach. Doctors or providers must be good coaches. Certainly, you may need medicines, radiation, surgery, or other procedures. All of those you clearly need, but don't forget your most important weapon: your brain and how you think. The state of your mind will be a critical weapon, maybe the most important of all. Positive thinking improves your immunity because neuropeptides, hormones, and neurotransmitters produced by the human brain affect the most important weapon of your immunity. It's a group effort. Dr. Lawrence LeShan proved scientifically that having a purpose in life could double the lifespan of a lot of his cancer patients, and it increased their spontaneous cure rate. As a psychiatrist, he treated his regular cancer patients for forty-five years. I lived within three blocks of the Metropolitan Museum of Art in New York City; that's why the following story of Dr. LeShan interested me a great deal. He had a female patient with metastatic breast cancer all over her body. His counseling session once a month with the patient was to take her to lunch at the Metropolitan Museum of Art. He then would walk her through the museum and they would look at her favorite art for thirty minutes. They did that for five years. She was restudied after that time and no cancer was found. There are many stories like this in his famous book. The information in this section will help you mobilize yourself and your healing abilities, and bring the power of your mind to the forefront. The medical profession in general has disconnected the brain from the human body. It started in 1635, when René Descartes gave the brain to the church and the body to science. We've been practicing like that for over three hundred years and it's slowly beginning to change. A famous book, *Descartes' Error*, was written about that. Thoughts and feelings do not cause or cure cancer, but they affect the body chemistry, our immunity, and can have a great effect on your illness. All of us destroy some cancer cells in our body every day; that is our immunity. The immune system is strongly affected by feelings, and it's a lack of immunity that causes a great deal of cancer. If immunity is down, viruses, bacteria, as well as cancer attack our bodies. If immunity is suppressed with steroids and a cancerous organ is transplanted by mistake, it will literally take over our body within days. That is in the medical literature. We live longer, maybe double the lifespan, and increase our spontaneous cures when we mobilize a compromised immune system. Dr. LeShan, in his famous and great book *Cancer As a Turning Point*, taught patients to mobilize this self-healing mechanism and brought it to the aid of scientific medical treatment. He tries to find out what his patients' purpose in life may be. It is interesting how he does that. He will ask the patient to tell him in five minutes what his or her purpose in life might be. He will say that a fairy godmother has come and will grant the patient any wish if he or she had five minutes to tell her what it is, and then he will work with the patient on it and try to achieve that dream. As mentioned already multiple times, your immunity is related to your thought process. Doctor LeShan was a psychotherapist with a lot of experience and this is the method he eventually ended up with after treating patients for many years. He always want to know what is right with you; how could he switch you to a creative path and not a destructive way of thinking. What kind of life would get you out of bed in the morning and lead you to purposeful work, make you happy and peaceful? What would give you the maximum zest and enthusiasm in life? He felt this was critical. What kind of life with creativity would make you happy? That is the road to healing.

# Beating Cancer with Nutrition

Sugar can have great influence on the progression or cause of cancer.

We've already learned that the hope, optimism, and fighting spirit have healing power. So does what we eat. Eating a nutrient-dense diet has great value. Be in the present moment, value your mission, know your purpose, cherish your friends and family, and savor sunsets and sunrises. Soak up music and laughter, and play the notes that uplift you. Be at peace with your creativity. Be enthusiastic. Cancer is a sugar feeder. Eat high-nutrient foods as described in my book, *The Secret of the Non Diet for Adults*, and by Dr. Joel Fuhrman in his book *Super Immunity*. Slow the growth for the cancer by not providing the sugary fuel. Exercise is great at burning fat and sugar in your muscles. That helps the fight against cancer. Make nutrient food your way of life. Eat low-glycemic-index (50 percent) complex carbohydrates, 100 percent whole grains, vegetables and legumes, and fruit—all you can eat!

Cancer is a wasting disease; 40 percent actually die from malnutrition. So eat a lot of high-nutrient foods. I myself eat a pile of food for lunch, but it is foods of color. I personally help design the doctors' lunches, except they don't know it. It's like trying to get your children to change the way they eat. Change your food a little at a time and don't even talk about it. The way to eat is: low-glycemic-index (less than 50 percent) complex carbohydrates, 100 percent whole grains, vegetables, beans, and all the fruit you can eat. You'll be very healthy and not feed the cancer. Visit www.glycemicindex.com for more information.

The backbone of the immune system is protein—protein from plants, without fat. If you can't eat solid foods, drink smoothies made from all sorts of fruits, adding flaxseed, vitamins, and protein powder if you wish. I have one of those every other day with oatmeal and fruit in between. A well-nourished cancer patient will have healthy cells again and avoid the toxicity of chemotherapy.

Your immune system consists of twenty trillion cells; the army, navy, and air force fighting the war for you. Eat well, take supplements, and lower your stress level. Your immunity is your lifeline; you must learn to use it. Eat foods as close to their natural state as possible and eat as many colorful vegetables as you can tolerate. If it doesn't rot or sprout, throw it out. Don't eat anything with a mother or a face—ha! Fish oil, flaxseed, multiple vitamins, and vitamin D are anti-inflammatory and helpful. The right fats, omega-3s, feed the beneficial prostaglandins, which are critical to beating cancer. Omega-3s improve the immune system and are more likely to destroy the cancer cells.

Nearly six hundred thousand people die from cancer each year. Nine hundred thousand or more are alive, and five hundred thousand are cured—not bad. There is great hope. Let's get you into the five hundred thousand. Respect your body, and fill your home with joy, passion, hopefulness, music, laughter, play, thankful friends, family, and work. There is no time or room for dying; you are too busy. Your body remembers what it's like to be well. There's a doctor living within you, the immune system. Your body knows how to repair itself. Cancer in a host is like a seed in the soil. Let's change the environment that it's growing in. The time has come to put major emphasis on the soil. What we need, how we exercise, and how we control our psychology are critical. Dr. John Grant has estimated that 40 percent or more of cancer patients die from malnutrition and not their cancer. Natural forces within us are the true healers.

Each patient carries his own doctor within him. Lifestyle is about 90 percent responsible for cancer, with your genetics accountable for about 10 percent at best, according to Dr. Patrick Quillin. He has written a great book, *Beating Cancer with Nutrition*, from which I'm quoting liberally. I highly recommend you read that book. Nutrition supports the immune system. Remember, sugar feeds cancer, which makes diet and antioxidant supplements critical. The earlier the patient receives nutrient therapy, the better the outcome. Nutrients can decrease the rate of cancer cell division, and can reverse the cancer cell to a healthy cell. It will greatly improve your immune system. Every cell in your body is eavesdropping on your thoughts. So how you think becomes critical in the fight against cancer. Sugar is the most dangerous chemical in your body when in excess. We need a certain amount of it for energy and brain function, but it is the excess of oxygen and sugar metabolism that produces free radicals which will promote cancer growth. Fructose is a lot healthier, has a low glycemic index of thirty, and promotes good health. The following are the three main reasons why excessive sugar is not good for cancer. Rises in blood glucose generate corresponding rises of insulin, which pushes prostaglandin production toward the immune system, suppressing PGE-2. While fish oil, EPA, and GLA have a favorable impact on cancer, these potent essential fatty acids are anti-inflammatory when blood levels are high. Secondly, cancer cells feed directly on blood glucose, like a fermenting yeast organism. A cancer patient eating sugar is like throwing gasoline on a smoldering fire. Thirdly, elevating glucose level suppresses the immune system. Cancer cells primarily use glucose for fuel, with lactic acid as a by-product.

# Nutrition and Diet

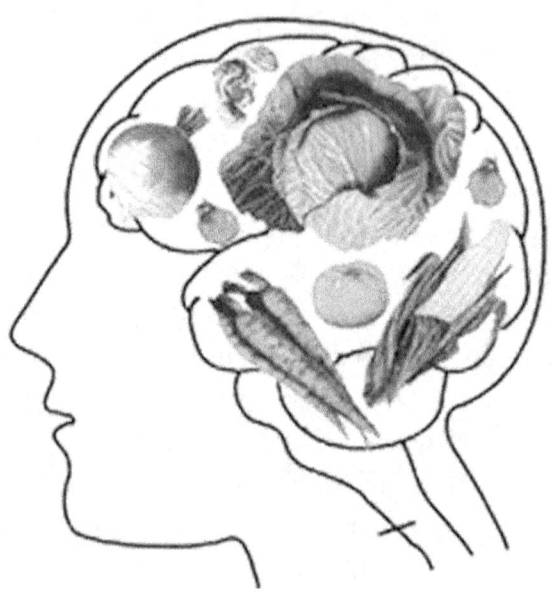

You always hear that diets don't work. I completely agree, but occasionally a person makes it by counting calories. Only a few people get away with that. Calories in are not calories out. Sorry. If you eat one hundred calories of fat, 97 percent sits on your abdomen or buttocks within four hours. Only 3 percent is used up in metabolism. Of each one hundred calories of low-glycemic-index foods, complex carbohydrates, only about 60 percent will ever enter your bloodstream because of fiber. Forty percent is used up in the metabolism because of the fiber of complex carbohydrates. So it is what you eat that counts, not calorie counting.

There are successful and unsuccessful dieters. Most are unsuccessful due to the type of food they are eating and the psychology of food. Remember, food is a drug and we have to use our brain as we eat every day. If you follow a strong program of proper food selection, I call that the non diet. I suggest you read the book I've written about this, *The Secret of the Non Diet.* There is one for children and one for adults. I follow a flexitarian diet, an 80 percent vegan way of eating: low-glycemic-index complex carbohydrates, 100 percent whole grains, and all-you-can-eat vegetables and fruit, essentially. I eat fish twice a week, no beef, and no dairy products. I teach this at my wellness centers. "Dr. Kachmann's Twelve-Week Weight Loss Program" is extremely successful.

Many of the clients in these classes tell me they like this program better than many other well-known programs, because I put a greater emphasis on the psychology of eating. I have heard that statement many times.

Many men and women are dissatisfied with their body size and shape. Men generally take up exercise to lose weight, but for women, body dissatisfaction translates into a diet.

As a wellness doctor and neurosurgeon, I have about two hundred people participating in my twelve-week weight loss program, and about 90 percent are women. The translation of body dissatisfaction into dieting is facilitated by the diet industry, which perpetuates the belief that thin is the desired state.

My wellness instructors and I teach from the standpoint of psychology and the total wellness picture. We talk a lot about stress and the mind-body diseases that it can cause. See the mind-body index for how to avoid vascular disease, strokes, heart attacks, cancer, immune diseases, and Alzheimer's disease. Some people call Alzheimer's disease type 3 diabetes. The major emphasis is on the reasons we are using food as a drug to calm our mind.

Dieting today aims to reduce food intake, or starve us, and cause weight loss. But research indicates that dieting causes episodes of overeating. Research has been inspired by the restraining theory and has highly dis-inhibited eating behavior as a consequence. We don't want to do it. Starvation is not associated with pleasure; it is the opposite of the survival mechanism. Everything necessary for our survival has pleasure associated with it: sex and food. Imposing cognitive limits on food intake is not popular.

Explanations of dis-inhibition include the rebound of overeating, which emphasizes the dieters' cognitive limits, a change in cognition and mood, and a paradoxical response to denial and escape theory, which highlights the role of self-awareness. Research has drawn parallels between eating behavior and addictive behavior (see the section on food addiction). Restricting the diet does not always lead to overeating. Some people can do it. Some diets are successful in the attempts to eat less, but this is only in a small number of people over a longer time. There a lot of people from Weight Watchers in my classes, for example, yet I have seen a number of people for whom it worked.

I definitely don't recommend the high-protein diets. I've read books that call them a fraud. Robert Atkins, author of the *Akins Diet* died at a fairly young age, when you restrict carbohydrates, you will have weight loss very quickly, because you are depleting the glycogen from your muscles. You have about three pounds of glycogen, and each carries with it about two to three pounds of water. You lose ten pounds in nothing flat. But then eventually you will get a ravenous appetite and eat more than ever. I've see that many times. Besides, the meat products you eat carry with them a lot of very unhealthy fat.

Many times, we feel dissatisfied with our body size and shape and this dissatisfaction results in one diet after another. I highly recommend following my book, *The Secret of the Non Diet*, with its food selection of low-glycemic complex carbohydrates, 100 percent whole grains, and all-you-can-eat vegetables and fruit; you will be just fine. If you have a serious illness like advanced heart disease or stroke, follow a very strict, high-nutrient-dense, vegan way of eating and you can change things around and save your life. It is well documented in many books. Look at the recommended books on my Web site, www.kachmannmindbody.com.

A diet is often sabotaged by the psychological consequences of imposing limits on food intake, and attempting to choose a healthy diet becomes more problematic. Of course, you must remember that overeating is associated with other problems, including obesity, and many diseases that can cause us great harm.

# Super Immunity – The Gold

The immune system—our army, navy, air force, and marines that defend our health—will determine our lifespan. Dr. Joel Fuhrman wrote a great book, *Super Immunity*, that was recently published. It really is the gold of longevity and health teaching. I read a preview copy twice and was asked by the publisher to write a few words about it. I think if you follow what is recommended, including the recipes in the back of the book, unless you fell out of an airplane you would have a 90 billion percent chance of living to be one hundred or older with a sound mind. It is all about a nutrient-dense way of eating in which you eat the right macronutrients and micronutrients, vitamins, minerals, complex carbohydrates, 100 percent whole grains, proteins, fats, and phytochemicals. That creates a strong immune system, one that prevents vascular disease, heart attacks, strokes, cancer, infections, autoimmune disease, etc.

The China Study conducted by Colin Campbell proved that certain foods could provide health promotion and disease protection benefits. The study was done a few decades ago, but a lot of this information has been known for thousands of years. Natural plants are complex packages of biologically active compounds. The term *phytochemicals*, which means "of plant chemicals," represents the thousands of plant source compounds that have profound effects on human health and immunity. Scientific discoveries have proven that the phytochemicals run the machinery of metabolism. They are the co-enzymes that run the chemical reactions of our body. Our food, in other words, can help or harm our immunity. We are what we eat. It determines resistance to disease and increases our longevity. The benefits of good eating habits have been largely ignored by 80 percent of the American people, who now are having a high incidence of illness, resulting in a lot of diseases, poor health, and tremendous cost. Koreans, Japanese, Micronesians, South Americans, and Africans are being devastated by the sad, mad, toxic diet of fat, salt, and sugar. The human body can take advantage of the complex biochemical compounds found in plants and use these to keep a normal weight, prevent illness, and heal previously damaged cells. We need to start paying attention to the defense and repair mechanism of our bodies. The twenty-five thousand phytochemicals are bioactive, plant-derived chemical compounds important for the growth and survival of the planet. The human immune system evolved dependent on the phytochemicals for its optimal functioning. The plants use these phytochemicals to defend themselves against their enemies—funguses, viruses, bacteria, and animals.

Superior nutrition is the secret of the "superior immunity" that Dr. Joel Fuhrman writes about. You don't have to be a genius to realize that. There is great synergism of the human immune system and the phytochemicals of our plants. Animal protein does not have the same synergism in the human body.

Animals and plants develop a fragile, interconnected, and symbiotic relationship on earth. Now human beings rely on plants for health and survival.

We are what we eat. We are made from what we eat. Fat, salt, and sugar are not going to do it for you. That's what 80 percent of Americans eat and look at the obesity rate—65 percent. One-third of children are overweight. When we cultivate nutritional deficiencies in our body over long periods of time, especially in our formative years, it creates a lot of cellular damage, resulting in serious illnesses later in life. Advancements in nutritional science have fostered an opportunity to create great health, increase longevity, and prevent disease, including cancer, heart attacks, and strokes, which are well known in vegetarian societies. The chemical compounds found in vegetables, beans, berries, and fruits, when combined with nuts, seeds, mushrooms, and onions, fuel the miraculous self-healing and self-protective properties already built into the human genome. The American diet is a disaster of processed foods and animal products which represent 85 percent of a mad, sad diet that is very low in natural vegetables and includes very few phytochemicals, and as a result the nutrients are dramatically deficient in plant-derived disease-fighting chemicals. Less than 10 percent of the foods we consume are unrefined foods. Ninety percent of our food has been stripped of healthy fiber. We are not eating enough fruits, beans, seeds, and vegetables. We are missing the beneficial antioxidants and phytochemicals that repair the body and prevent disease. The carotene family (alpha and beta), lutein, zeaxanthin, lycopene, flavonoids, alphalipoic acid, quercetin, anthocyanins, ligands, pectins, etc., are among the great chemicals that can heal us and prevent cancer and numerous inflammatory diseases, and are found in the vegetables and beans we eat. Since neither processed foods nor animal products contain a significant load of antioxidant nutrients and phytochemicals, the modern diet is dramatically prone to disease.

Antioxidants are vitamins, minerals, and phytochemicals that aid the body in removing free radicals, which cause disease and can kill us. The vast majority of antioxidants are made available to the body through our consumption of fruits, vegetables, and other natural plants. Oxidative damage occurs when free radical activity in the body increases and free radicals burst out of their cellular compartments to affect broader regions of the cells. Vegetables are so rich in antioxidant chemical compounds that eating a vegetarian, vegan, or nutritarian diet is an easy way to increase the antioxidant capacity. Foods with great amounts of phytochemicals are cabbage, red peppers, carrots, green peppers, tomatoes, onions, broccoli, peas, squash, and mushrooms. A phytochemical-deficient diet is responsible for a weak immune system, resulting in disease and death at a young age. Populations with much higher amounts of vegetables in their diet have 50 to 70 percent lower rates of cancer and inflammatory diseases. The longest-living populations throughout history are the ones with a high intake of vegetables in their diet. Dr. Joel Fuhrman says that the phytochemicals are the most important discovery in human nutrition during the last fifty years. The concentration of phytochemicals is often highlighted by vibrant colors of black, blue, red, green, and orange—except maybe for the very healthy mushrooms.

The benefits of phytochemicals are:
- Detoxifying enzymes
- Controlling the production of free radicals
- Deactivation and detoxification of cancer-producing agents
- Protecting cell structure from damage by toxins
- Fueling mechanisms to repair damaged DNA
- Introducing beneficial antifungal, antibacterial, and antiviral effects
- Inhibiting the function of damaged or genetically altered DNA
- Improving function of immune cells
- Producing great disease-fighting antibodies—preventing cancer

## The War on Cancer

Our cancer rates exploded between 1935 and 2005. There has been an increasing rate every year, for seventy years. We've had an explosion of immune system dependent diseases, allergies, autoimmune disease, and cancer.

Cruciferous vegetables are great anticancer agents. Green vegetables such as kale, cabbage, broccoli, cauliflower, and turnips are called cruciferous because as a flower they have four petals arranged like a cross. Cruciferous vegetables have a unique chemical composition. They make a sulfur containing compound, where the cells are programmed to release ITCs, an array of compounds with proven powerful immune-boosting effects in anticancer activity. Eating cruciferous vegetables, chewing them and breaking down the cellular structure, decreases cancer rates dramatically. Consuming mushrooms regularly is associated with a significant decrease in the risk of breast cancer. Frequent consumption of mushrooms can decrease the incidence of breast cancer 60 to 70 percent. So, what's the solution? Dr. Fuhrman has a great formula: H=N/C. Health expectancy equals nutrient density divided by calories. There is our destiny.

To slow the aging process we need to eat the nutrient-dense diet, essentially all-you-can-eat vegetables, beans, and fruits. Counting calories or portion control is not needed if you eat nutrient-dense foods.

Dr. Fuhrman's diet in his book *Eat to Live*:
- Vegetable based
- Lots of fruits and beans
- Seeds and nuts
- Oil used sparingly
- Animals products zero to three times a week

The standard American diet:
- Grain based
- Lots of dairy and meat
- Lots of oil
- Major animal products five to seven times a week
- Focus on nutrient-poor calories

## *The Gold*

Resistant starches means starches with a lot of fiber. The starchy foods will not be all absorbed because of high fiber content. At least 30 to 40 percent of calories are lost in metabolism. They never enter the bloodstream. The starch from a baked potato will have a high absorption rate because of lack of fiber. Calories in and calories out, the original concept, was incorrect. Beans promote a sensation of fullness. They improve insulin sensitivity, decreasing diabetes. Beans promote good bacteria once the bowel adjusts. Beans also have in them a lot of good essential fatty acids, which you need. The carbohydrates in them have a lot of fiber and not all will be absorbed, and you can eat a lot of them because of that.

- Black beans – 63 percent fiber
- Red kidney beans – 56 percent fiber
- Navy beans – 52 percent fiber
- Lentils – 47 percent fiber
- Split peas – 38 percent fiber
- Corn – 32 percent fiber

The high-nutrient-dense diet will enhance cellular repair mechanisms and reverse disease. That is why the way of eating that Dr. Dean Ornish recommends for preventing, stopping, and reversing heart disease works. He essentially teaches the same thing as myself and Dr. Fuhrman. This way of eating reduces the inflammatory response, suppresses genetic alterations, decreases free radical activity, slows the metabolic rate, enhances DNA repair, and removes toxins.

# Nutrition and Nuts

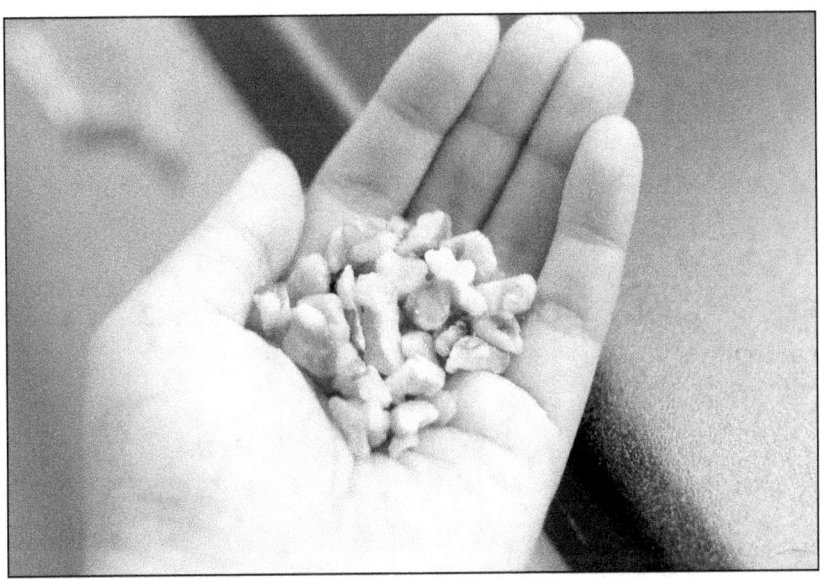

Dr. Dean Ornish published many papers and books long ago by proving that most disease is preventable, stoppable, and reversible by proper food selection, exercise, and stress reduction. Seldom do I meet a cardiologist that has read his work. Type 2 diabetes, vascular disease, heart attacks, strokes, and cancer are diet diseases at least 90 percent of the time. So what should we be doing? The cardiologist or medical oncologist should meet you with diet book or DVDs in hand, or provide a set program you must participate in and follow up to encourage you to do it. I have faith in you; it can be done.

I encourage you to read the works of Dr. Dean Ornish.

Dr. Esselstyn from the Cleveland Clinic ran a large study of patients with advanced vascular disease and type 2 diabetes, and proved that proper food selection and exercise had a huge effect on the patients he worked with. They will all live twenty years longer. Don't you think we should pay attention to that? He also promotes a plant-based diet like what I teach at my Mind-Body Institute.

Incidentally, lean meats are not your friend, either. They still have a lot of fat. It's easier to exclude fat when you don't eat animal products. If you're having trouble making a decision about that, think of the torture they had to go through before they landed on the table. I once read a description of that in one of Dr. Robin Cook's mystery books and I never ate a hamburger again.

A pure vegan diet over twelve weeks will result in weight loss, as well as a change in your food preferences and your taste buds. You will then be on the way to a low-fat plant-based diet. If you having great results, you can always backslide 10 to 20 percent, but initially I would go 100 percent.

Most foods from plants are low-fat, but exceptions are:
- Avocados
- Olives
- Nuts and seeds
- Some soy products

So keep them to a minimum, although eating one to two ounces of seeds and nuts is a good idea. Keep vegetable oil low because it is 100 percent fat. Use one tablespoon of olive oil; it's 120 calories.

We need to appreciate the power of the reproductive vehicles of plant production, nuts and seeds. They carry the genetic material, but are full of healthy essential fats, proteins, vitamin E, and minerals. Eating nuts and seeds increases the phytochemical absorption of green leafy vegetables at least ten times, according to Dr. Joel Fuhrman.

Nuts and seeds have increased oil content, but mainly the monounsaturated and polyunsaturated fats, which are much healthier for you—not the saturated fats of animal meats.

What's a health nut? A person that exercises hard and watches what he eats.

There are more than three hundred kinds of nuts. As you know, each plant has a seed, but only a few are used for food. After all, we have over one hundred thousand types of plants. Peanuts by far are the most common seeds eaten in the U.S., and account for approximately 70 percent of production.

You would think the overeating of nuts and seeds would lead to obesity, but a population study of twenty-five thousand Americans found that people who consumed the most nuts were less obese. An explanation may be that they turn the appetite down for a period. I found that to be true. I keep some in my car, and when I'm getting hungry I eat about ten of them, and ten minutes later my appetite has lessened. I highly recommend eating six to ten nuts about an hour before dinner, and you will eat a lot less.

Nuts produce a chemical called arginine, which is thought to dilate blood vessels and therefore helps prevent vascular disease. Also, the nurses' health study, the physicians' health study, and the Iowa women's health study found nut consumption is linked to a low risk of heart disease. It perhaps reduces it as much as 30 percent.

Some think that fat from nuts is a good substitute for the saturated fats of meat and dairy. The reduction of vascular disease is as high as 45 percent. This includes reduction in risk of cancer, dementia, and autoimmune diseases.

The reduction in type 2 diabetes may be related to improvement in cell membrane metabolism. It reduces insulin resistance that causes type 2 diabetes.

Nuts are commonly used to make oils. Remember, all vegetable oils are 100 percent fat, but some have medicinal and cosmetic purposes. They are used commonly in salad dressings, baking, and cooking. So look out for them; you may have a healthy salad in front of you, but are killing it with vegetable oils. Some oils are healthier than others. Macadamia nut, coconut, sesame, and canola oils are more stable than the others and it is more difficult to break them down into trans-fats.

Canola oil is made from rapeseeds with the toxic erucic acid removed. It has gained great popularity as being safer than olive oil for general use. It has a high percentage of omega-3, the good essential fat.

Highly polyunsaturated oils such as flaxseed and sunflower are not recommended if they're going to be exposed to heat, because heat changes the chemical structure of the fatty acids and forms free radicals. These oils are best used for salad dressing. Other oils are best avoided.

Cottonseed oil may contain toxic residues from spraying the fields. Flaxseed or black currant oils are the most popular. Flaxseed is probably the safest, because it has a high omega-3 content and is less expensive.

Nuts and seeds are best stored in the shell. Shells protect them from free radical damage. Shelled nuts should be refrigerated. Nuts and seeds improve food flavor and improve metabolism of the rest of the food ten times.

Remember, there are many safety issues with nuts and seeds because of allergies. One percent of the U.S. population has nut and seed allergies, and they can be very serious. Nut allergies tend to be fixed and don't change.

Some nuts, such as almonds and walnuts, are very low in cholesterol, but are high in monounsaturated and polyunsaturated fat—the good fats. One to two ounces a day of nuts are recommended. Add some to your oatmeal and salads.

### Almonds

In the United States, almonds are grown only in California. They have a 60 percent fat content and a high caloric content, but they are full of nutrients. Three and a half ounces of almonds have six hundred calories, so limit the amount, but definitely eat them if you're not allergic. They're full of monounsaturated and polyunsaturated fats, which you need. They are 20 percent protein, and have potassium, magnesium, calcium, iron, zinc, vitamin E, antioxidants, and flavonoids. They are an anticancer food. One-third cup of shelled almonds contains 280 calories, twenty-four grams of fat, nine grams of protein, and ten grams of carbohydrate. They lower LDL and raise HDL cholesterol.

## Cashews

Cashew nuts are a well-known kidney-shaped nut. They are the seeds at the bottom of the cashew apple, and light-colored and delicate in flavor. They are the favored nuts of Dr. Joel Fuhrman. Cashews are second in fat to almonds. They are a good source of monounsaturated fats, minerals, magnesium, potassium, iron, and zinc, and well as biotin and protein. One-third cup has approximately 260 calories, twenty-one grams of protein, and fifteen grams of carbohydrate. They are low in fat content and high in protein compared to most other nuts. They are 65 percent fat, but it is mainly omega-3.

## Chestnuts

Enclosed in glossy, soft, mahogany-colored shells, chestnuts are seeds of the chestnut tree. They're the size of a walnut, are low in fats, are primarily carbohydrate, and have a lot of vitamin C, which other nuts don't have. They are a good source of minerals.

# Nutrition and Grains

"Whole grain" means the grain has all three of its original elements.

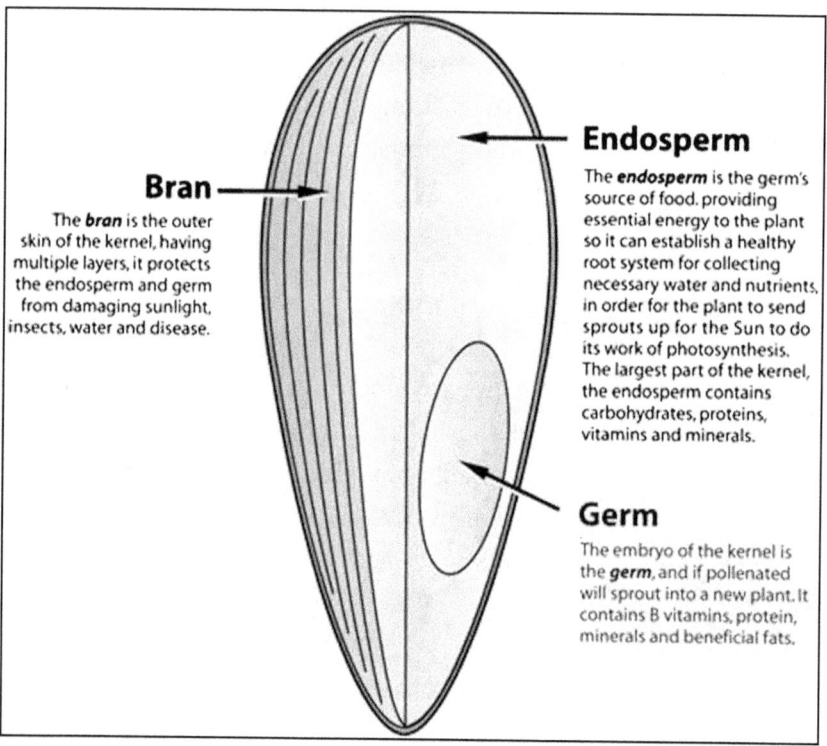

**Bran**

The **bran** is the outer skin of the kernel, having multiple layers, it protects the endosperm and germ from damaging sunlight, insects, water and disease.

**Endosperm**

The **endosperm** is the germ's source of food. providing essential energy to the plant so it can establish a healthy root system for collecting necessary water and nutrients, in order for the plant to send sprouts up for the Sun to do its work of photosynthesis. The largest part of the kernel, the endosperm contains carbohydrates, proteins, vitamins and minerals.

**Germ**

The embryo of the kernel is the **germ**, and if pollenated will sprout into a new plant. It contains B vitamins, protein, minerals and beneficial fats.

The outer shell or bran contains the fiber and vitamin B. The germ contains phytochemicals and vitamin B. The endosperm contains the carbohydrates and protein.

The key is the grain is whole and not refined by stripping away the bran and the germ, leaving only the endosperm. The whole grain should be left intact—meaning you get more fiber and more micronutrients—raising the blood sugar and resultant insulin level less and reducing their caloric intake through metabolism. Remember that with fiber a lot of the calories are not metabolized.

## *Fake-out Words*

- Made with: maybe just a drop of whole wheat
- One hundred percent wheat: some are a lot, yes, or no whole wheat
- Multi-grain: tells you nothing about whether they are whole wheat or refined
- Blends: "whole grain blend" probably has little whole grain
- Supports heart health: this means little
- Good source: means eight grams of whole grain, 15 percent
- Excellent source: sixteen grams of whole grain, 27 percent

To make sure you receive the health and dietary benefits of whole grain and wheat, the label should read 100 percent whole grain or 100 percent whole wheat. That way, you avoid the refined flour, high fructose corn syrup, and added sugar.

## *What Is a Nutritarian?*

A nutritarian is a person whose food choices are influenced by nutritional quality, who strives for more micronutrients per calorie in the diet, and who recognizes that food is a powerful disease fighter for an effective and therapeutic effect. Nuts and seeds are good for weight loss. They have a lot of fiber in them and carry a lot of good essential fatty acids. You should eat at least one ounce a day. A lot of people get away with two ounces because nuts decrease the appetite tremendously.

How do you prevent, stop, and reverse vascular disease and diabetes?

- Eat at least fifty grams of fiber daily
- Eat a 20 percent fat diet; fat from seeds, nuts, and vegetables
- Eat sufficient omega-3, the essential fatty acids
- Eat a high phytochemical and antioxidant diet
- Low-glycemic-index foods
- Low-calorie, dense foods
- Minimal animal products; two to three servings a week

## IGF

High levels of the hormone IGF reduce longevity and lead to cancer. Low levels lead to increased lifespan and decrease inflammation, decrease oxidative damage, increase insulin sensitivity, and slow the aging process. The amount of meat we eat determines the IGF level, which is almost totally dependent on our animal meat consumption. We have at least twenty major recommendations to follow in order to live to be a hundred and be of sound mind. But, what to eat by far will have the greatest effect. Your food selection is critical to your longevity.

# Motivation and Self-Esteem

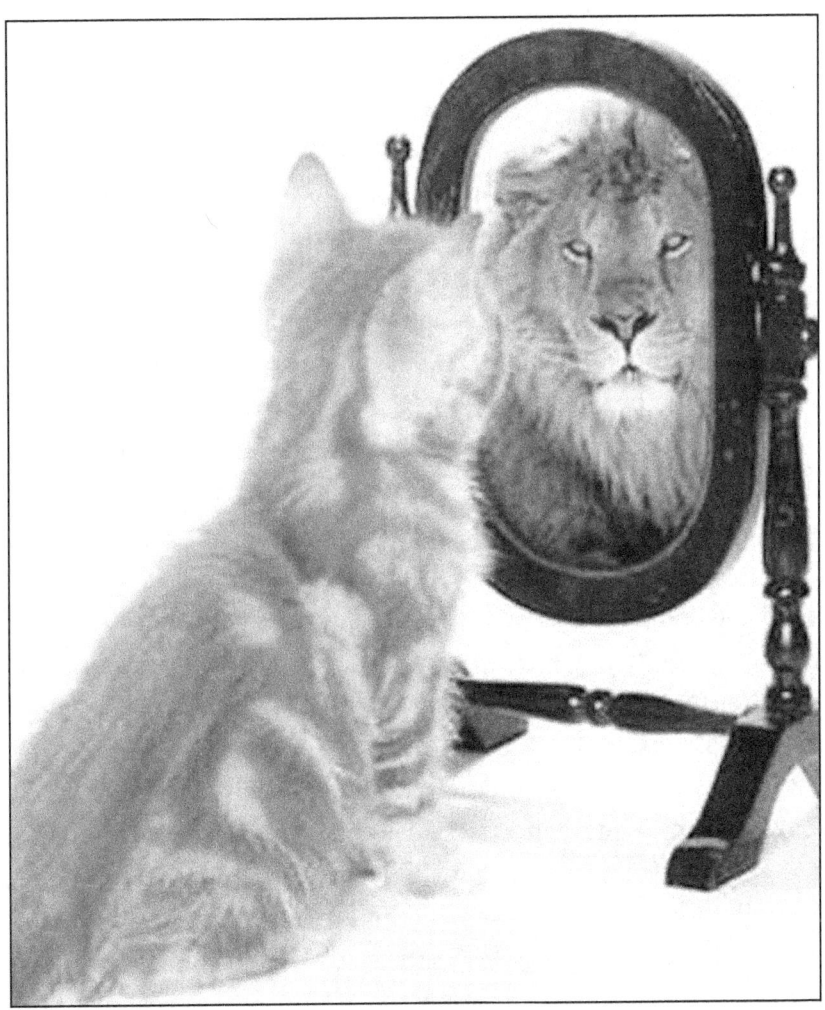

Self-esteem is a fundamental human need. Without it, it is difficult to motivate ourselves. It works its way within us, with or without our knowledge. Self-esteem, fully realized, is the experience that we are appropriate to life and to its requirements. Self-esteem is confidence in our ability to think and to cope with the basic challenges of life; confidence in our right to be successful and happy. It is the feeling of being worthy, deserving, entitled to assert our needs and wants, achieve our values, and enjoy the fruits of our efforts. Self-esteem represents an achievement, a reward for work activities.

The power of one's conviction about oneself lies in the fact that one is more than a judgment or a feeling. It is a motivator. It inspires behavior. It is directly affected by how we act. There is a continuous feedback loop between our actions in the world and our self-esteem. The level of our self-esteem influences how we act, and how we act influences the level of our self-esteem. To trust one's mind and to know that one is worthy of happiness is the essence of self-esteem. If I trust my mind in judgment, I am more likely to operate as a thinking being. By exercising my ability to think and bringing appropriate awareness to my activities, my life works better. This reinforces trust in my mind. and I am more likely to be mentally positive and bring more awareness to my activities and more persistence to solve problems. I feel justified in distrusting my mind—the opposite of self-esteem. With high self-esteem, I am more likely to be justified in trusting my mind in the face of difficulties. With low self-esteem, I am more likely to give up, or go through the motions of trying without really giving it my best. High self-esteem subjects were more persistent people. If I persevere, the likelihood is that I will succeed more often than I will fail.

If I respect myself and require that others deal with me respectfully, I send out signals and behave in ways that increase the likelihood that others will respond appropriately. If I lack self-respect and consequently accept discourtesy, abuse, or exploitation from others as natural, I unconsciously transmit this, and somebody will treat me at my self-estimate. When this happens and I submit to it, my self-respect deteriorates still more. The value of self-esteem lies in the fact that it not only allows us to feel better, but it allows us to live better, to respond to challenges and opportunities more resourcefully and appropriately.

The level of our self-esteem has profound consequences for every aspect of our existence: how we operate in the workplace, how we deal with people, how likely we are to rise in the company, what we plan to achieve, how we interact with our spouse, children, and friends—our level of personal happiness. Healthy self-esteem correlates with rationality, realism, creativity, independence, flexibility, ability to manage change, willingness to admit mistakes, benevolence, and cooperativeness. Poor self-esteem correlates with irrationality, blindness to reality, rigidity, fear of the new and unfamiliar, inappropriate conformity or inappropriate rebelliousness, defensiveness, overly compliant or controlling behavior, and fear of or hostility toward others.

High self-esteem seeks to channel and stimulate worthwhile and demanding goals. A rich set of goals nurtures good self-esteem. Low self-esteem seeks the safety of the familiar and undemanding. Confining oneself to this serves to weaken self-esteem.

The more solid our self-esteem, the better equipped we are to cope with troubles that arise in our personal lives or in our careers; the quicker we are to pick ourselves up after a fall, the more energy we have to begin anew. Most successful people have had a number of failures, but they dust themselves off and start again with enthusiasm. The higher our self-esteem, the more ambitious we tend to be, not necessarily in a career, but in terms of what we hope to experience of life—emotionally, intellectually, creatively, and spirituality. The lower our self-esteem, the less we aspire to and the less we are likely to achieve. Either path tends to be self-reinforcing and self-perpetuating.

The higher our self-esteem, the stronger the drive to express ourselves, reflecting the spirituality within us. The higher our self-esteem, the more open, honest, and appropriate our communications are likely to be, because we believe our thoughts have value and therefore we welcome all the interior clarity. The lower our self-esteem, the more evasive and inappropriate our communications are likely to be, because of uncertainty about our own thoughts and feelings and/or anxiety about the listless response. The higher our self-esteem, the more disposed we are to form nourishing rather than toxic relationships. We tend to feel most comfortable, most at home with persons whose self-esteem level resembles our own.

What is required for many of us is the courage to tolerate happiness without self-sabotage. Prejudging is a sign of poor self-esteem, and the need to perceive some other group as inferior. Self-esteem, high or low, tends to be a generator of self-fulfilling prophecies. We function better with self-esteem and it is a basic need in all of us. It is an essential contribution to the life process. It is indispensable to normal and healthy development; it has survival value. An excess of troubles can surely knock down people with high self-esteem, but they're quicker to pick themselves up.

Good self-esteem increases the likelihood that we will find a way to meet our everyday needs. Good self-esteem has economic value. If we lack adequate self-esteem, the amount of choice offered to us today can be frightening.

Self-esteem has two interrelated components. One is a sense of basic confidence in the face of life's challenges—self-efficacy. The other is a sense of being worthy of happiness—self-respect. Self-efficacy needs confidence in the functioning of my mind; in my ability to think, understand, learn, choose, and make decisions; confidence in my ability to understand the facts of reality that fall within my interests and needs; self-trust and self-reliance. Self-respect means assurance of my value, and my strong attitude toward my right to live and be happy; comfort in properly asserting thoughts, wants, and needs; the feeling that joy and fulfillment are my natural birthright. Self-esteem is the disposition to experience oneself as confident, able to cope with the basic challenges of life, and to be worthy of happiness.

Self-esteem is a basic need. Our need for self-esteem is the result of two basic facts, both intrinsic to our species. The first is that we depend on it for survival in our successful mastery of the environment and the appropriate use of our consciousness, life and well-being, and ability to think. The second is that the right use of our consciousness is not automatic, is not wired in by nature. In the regulating of its activity, there is a crucial element of choice, therefore, of personal responsibility. Our survival and well-being depends on the guidance of our distinctive form of consciousness, the form uniquely human; our conceptual faculty, the faculty of abstraction, generalization, and integration. In other words, how we think is everything; we are dependent on our mind.

Human essence it is our ability to reason, which means to grasp relationships. It is on this ability, ultimately, that all life depends. It includes the totality of mental life, including the subconscious, the intuitive, and the symbolic comment, all of which are associated with the right brain. The mind is the means by which we reach out to and apprehend the world. We are the one species that can formulate a vision of what values are worth pursuing, and then pursue the opposite. If we have good self-esteem, we are more likely to make good choices. Look at the choices we have: focusing versus non-focusing, thinking versus non-thinking, awareness versus unawareness, respect for our reality versus avoidance of reality, respect of facts versus indifference to facts, respect for truth versus rejection of truth, honesty versus dishonesty.

The term *self-efficacy* is a basic power or confidence that we associate with healthy self-esteem, and *self-respect* to the experience of dignity and personal worth. To be efficacious is to be capable of producing a desired result. Confidence in a basic efficacy is the confidence and ability to learn what we need to learn and to do what we need to do in order to achieve our goals, insofar as success depends on our own efforts. Self-efficacy is the conviction that we can never make an error if we are able to think, to judge, to know, and to correct errors. It is trust in mental processes and abilities. In a world in which the total human knowledge is doubling about every ten years, our security rests only on our ability to learn. The root of self-efficacy is a home environment sufficiently sane, rational, and predictable as to allow us to believe understanding is possible, that thinking is not futile. As far as our own actions are concerned, the root is the will, efficacy itself, a refusal to surrender to helplessness, and the quest to understand even in the face of difficulties.

Self-respect entails expectation of friendship, love, and happiness as natural, as a result of who we are and what we do. A concern with right and wrong is not merely the product of social conditioning. A concern with morality or ethics arises naturally in the early stages of human development. The concept comes from adults, from whom you hear the words *good, bad, right,* and *wrong.* But the need is inherent in our nature. It is tied to the issue of survival. To be right as a person is to be fit for success and happiness; to be wrong is to be threatened by pain. The need for self-respect is basic and inescapable, inherent in our existence and humanity. Pride is the emotional reward for achievement; it is not a vice to be overcome by the value to be attained.

Self-esteem expresses itself in the face, manner, and way of talking and moving that projects the pleasure one takes in being alive. It expresses itself in the comfort one experiences in giving and receiving compliments, expressions of affection, appreciation, and the like. It expresses itself in an attitude of openness and a curiosity about new ideas, new experiences, and new possibilities in life. High self-esteem is intrinsically reality oriented. You have a respect for facts, and recognition of what is and what it is not. You cannot change what you wish to change unless you have a realistic outlook. Face it with good self-esteem and develop a program to change. Persons with high self-esteem have creativity, are able to manage change, have independence, have some flexibility, and have a willingness to admit and correct mistakes. Low self-esteem is associated with fear of reality. To change requires taking a realistic look at the present situation. Then you can be motivated to make the appropriate corrections.

## Stress and Cancer

Dr. Hans Selye from Canada published a great deal on the effects of stress on the body, both of animals and of humans. The doctor developed reticulum cell sarcoma, a type of cancer with a cure rate that is very low. This is the ultimate stress. Dr. Seley survived the cancer. He wasn't totally convinced of the relationship of cancer and the mind. He said, "All I can say as a scientist is that the great majority of physical illness have in part some psychological origin." Evidence gathered since he wrote those words suggests he was overly cautious. Dr. Seley's work was in the 1950s. The onset and continuation of a person's illness are strongly linked to a person's ability and willingness to deal with stress.

Stress that we choose evokes a response that is different from the stresses we like to avoid but cannot. Helplessness and hopelessness are worse than the stress itself. This is probably why cancer rates are higher among the economically deprived than the more well-to-do. Cancers are related to grief and depression.

Heart attacks occurred less commonly to type A personalities, who are in charge and more in control of their lives than their employees, who have less control and are subject to "deadly boredom." Stress comes mainly from the patient's interpretation of events.

Poverty, bereavement, and alcoholism are not stressful unless interpreted as such, and then will have their effects on a person's health. The scientific mind is rarely satisfied by some psychological studies in humans; there are too many variables. In mice, studies proved the cancer rate is 10 to 90 percent depending on the stress level—very interesting.

Cultures that place increased value on a combination of individual positive accomplishments are the most stressful. Societies with the least stress have the lowest rate of cancer. Close-knit communities in which support, loving relationships, and religious faith are the norm have a low cancer rate.

In some communities in India, with a pollution-free environment, a wholesome natural diet, relaxed yet strenuous work in the fields, dancing and storytelling, and plenty of rest, cancer is almost unknown. Those structured societies, when everyone knows his or her role, have less cancer. Mormons and Seventh-Day Adventists are examples.

Stress can be measured. Dr. Thomas Holmes and Dr. Rahe developed a stress test and it is readily available. The higher your number, the more mind-body illnesses, including cancer, you have. It's been scientifically proven.

Loss of a spouse is highest on the list. I've seen it many times among patients. Research has shown that within one day of any uncontrolled stress, the effectiveness of the immune system declines. People going through a divorce have a higher rate of cancer and heart disease. Married men have one-third the cancer rate of single men. Losing one's job or career increases the rate of cancer many times. Children with cancer have twice the amount of crises in the family. Another study revealed that thirty-one of thirty-three children with cancer had experienced a major loss within years of it occurring. How you cope is the answer; how you interpret the event is critical. If you live with it, control your feelings, don't become depressed, and control your stress, you may stay well. Depression involves giving up hope, and negative thinking is destructive. You're going on strike from life, losing interest. Hopelessness and helplessness lead to mind-body illnesses and cancer. Depression is a partial surrender to death and it is expressed at the cellular level. We literally speak to our seventy trillion body cells through hormones, neurotransmitters, and neuropeptides. Dr. Candace Pert proved that in her famous book *Molecules of Emotion*. Visualization and imaging does not work in people who deny their illness, because they don't connect to it and don't really participate in fighting it. If you don't mobilize your immune system with your mind it will not work. Psychiatrist Dr. George Engel concludes if he has patients draw pictures of their disease then it expresses their subconscious mind and you may find out the real truth of it. In the hopeless patient who doesn't want to participate in his or her treatment, he finds despair, anger, helplessness, hopelessness, and depression—a sure road to disaster. Many men die or develop cancer within six months after losing their job or retiring. They've lost their purpose in life. Men are more tied to their work. Men are better able to express anger, whereas women become depressed instead. Lack of an emotional outlet is common in the cancer patient. That is why cancer is more frequent in convents than in prisons. Fatalism can be fatal. A hopeless, helpless mother produces a hopeless, helpless child, and cancer may follow in either.

## Does Your Mind Target Organs in Your Body?

Psychological factors in the formative years of your life play a large part in where you will develop an illness if it occurs. It often determines what disease will occur in men and where it will appear. Target organs, just like in most mind-body illnesses, have special significance to the hormones, neurotransmitters, and neuropeptides made in your brain and your immune system. I see this all the time in my practice. At least 75 percent of the patients I see have some form of a mind-body illness related to their thought process. All our organs have receptor sights attached to their cells. Dr. Candace Pert was the first to prove that. The nerves of receptors vary from organ to organ. The bowel has four hundred thousand neuro cells. The heart has forty thousand neuro cells. The skin is our largest organ. The receptors have a "memory" in them. How many times have they been used by our neuropeptides, hormones, and neurotransmitters? So, abnormal cancer cells are more likely to attack or start in an organ's history.

# Is There a Psychological Profile of Cancer?

As far back as Galen in the second century AD, melancholy (depression) in people was more likely to lead to cancer than those with happiness and love in their life. In the eighth and ninth centuries, physicians realized that cancer tends to follow tragedy in a person's life, especially if his or her reaction was depression. Twentieth-century technological medicine has been reluctant to study the subject to develop a better understanding of the relationship of stress and cancer. It's a hard subject to study and difficult to develop control groups of different mind-sets, so the lack of interest is almost understandable. A book published in 1926, *A Psychological Study of Cancer* by Dr. Elida Evans, was largely ignored. It was only checked out six times from the Yale medical school library, according to Dr. Bernie S. Siegel. This book clearly spells out the cancer risk incurred by personality types for whom life's meaning comes entirely from people far outside the self. When that connection was disrupted, cancer followed in a high percentage of the people. It was well documented in this study. Cancer is a symbol of something wrong in the patient's life, a warning to take another road.

The typical cancer patient is characterized by, say, a man who expresses a lack of closeness to his parents, or a lack of unconditional love in childhood, or one who is not assured of his intrinsic value and ability to overcome challenges. As he grows up, he becomes extroverted and dependent on others for his self-esteem. Difficulty in forming more than superficial relationships leads to excruciating loneliness, according to Dr. LeShan, Dr. Evans, and Dr. Bernie Siegel. All have published great books on the subject. The truth is that generous, compulsive people who put others ahead of their own needs predominate among cancer patients. It's a disease of nice people. They are giving only to receive love that may be lacking in their lives Tests have been developed to help predict a psychological cancer profile. Dr. Bernie Siegel, from many years of experience, felt he could predict cancer by talking to a patient and getting to know him or her—interesting. Large studies going on for decades found the psychological profile that results in suicide, and not surprisingly, it was the same psychological setup that produces cancer.

# The Healing

So the job of the physician is to give the right medication and treatments, but also to discover the inner conflict and help the patient to resolve it. You need to know the patient and his psychological makeup. Unfortunately, in medicine today that is largely ignored. It is ignored in all aspects, but it is even more critical in the cancer patient. Their lives are dependent, and a large proportion of the time the physician needs to discover the reason for living. The human mind is incredibly powerful and it takes an equally powerful physician to turn it on. People who wish to get well with God alone or with the doctor alone, are minimizing their chances, it takes God and the doctor. Some would say there are no incurable diseases, only incurable people.

# The Will to Live Revisited

At first, the diagnosis of cancer may be heeded by a sense of denial. This allows a person to accept it over a period of time. Some don't believe it at all. A small number become psychologically unable to accept it and deny it forever and die. Knowing the truth but refusing to admit it would not lead to healing. Sharing one's fear and acting on it leads to the healing. Cancer is not a death sentence, but just a word. In his famous book, *The Will To Live*, Norman Cousins wrote: "The will to live is not a theoretical question but a physiological reality with consequences." How we speak to our seventy trillion body cells is critical in the healing. Dr. Bernie Siegel would ask his patient a number of questions, like, "Do you want to live to be a hundred?" Interestingly enough, when I give a lot of my mind-body lectures, I say, "I'm trying to get you to live to be a hundred with great health and a sound mind!" The second question he asked was, "How was life to you in the last year or two, before your illness?" Again, this relates to how I deal with patients. I always ask, "What's going on in your life?" rather than, "Where do you hurt?" This leads to the Holmes-Rahe test, the questionnaire to determine cancer and stress predisposition. The higher the number, the higher the chances are of you being a stressful person who developed mind-body illnesses, which include cancer. I designed the mind-body index and cancer is in it. Thirdly, what does the illness mean to you? What is your vision of the future? Do you want to see your children graduating, married, perhaps the birth of a grandchild? Would you have a purpose in life—finishing a novel, developing a new hobby? Fourthly, why do you need this illness? Maybe you're just tired of a meaningless life and need to turn in a different direction. Maybe you'll be forced to do that, or have the opportunity to do what you could not do on your present path. We cannot force people to change; we can only help them to change themselves. That is my experience in my forty-two years of medical practice, and it is very important to remember at times. Dr. Siegel believes all illnesses are psychosomatic; so do many others. I believe 75 percent of them are. That's why I formed the mind-body index.

# Importance of the Unconscious Mind

I believe the mind and body constantly communicate with each other. Candace Pert, in her famous book *Molecules of Emotion*, proved it in the '70s. The patient may express the will to live, but is it the truth? Dreams and images from the unconscious mind are more likely to tell the truth. Dr. Young, Sigmund Freud's pupil, felt it was too complicated and difficult to consistently determine the true motivation in a person's brain on a day-to-day basis. But these images are dreams that do indeed occur spontaneously and we need to take advantage of that. Images can be brought out through drawings and art. Art is commonly used in cancer therapy. It was especially used by Dr. Bernie Siegel. He could learn a great deal by interpreting art that a cancer patient had drawn for him. You have to be reborn as a new person; you need to develop a true will to live, a purpose in life to heal yourself. The best and easiest way to learn the patient's subconscious mind is by asking him or her to draw pictures. You should avoid excess verbal deception and get to the universal language of the unconscious mind. What you say can be a cover-up. When we communicate in visual images we are more likely to tell the truth. Imaging and visualization is the language of the unconscious mind. Analysis of the drawings is one of the doctor's most accurate aides to prognosis. Blood chemistry tells the present, drawings tell the future. By looking at their drawings, one researcher thought he could predict with 90 percent accuracy who would die within two months.

# Minimizing Side Effects of Chemo

Studies have shown that patients may be taking only 60 percent of the recommended chemotherapy drugs because of the fear of side effects:

change of appearance, loss of hair, weight loss, lack of energy, etc. Dr. Bernie Siegel believes 75 percent of the side effects of chemotherapy and radiation are caused by the patient's belief—a huge statistic. A lot of these reactions are induced by the negative, or nocebo, talk of the health-care providers. A better statement would be, "A lot of good things can happen between the treatments." It's much more empowering. Negative talk is the reason 25 percent of the patients start vomiting before the drugs are even given. One study revealed that when the patients were given only saline and not the chemo, 25 percent lost hair anyway, clearly proving the above.

## Avoiding the Voodoo Effect

The nocebo plays a huge part in medicine. We nocebo people (speak to them about the negative) all day long just by what we say. We use the CT scans, MRI scans, angiograms, X-rays, and plain old words to convince people that their symptoms are related to those studies. Sometimes that is the case; a lot of the time it may not be, intentional or unintentional. We say that the degenerative disease is the cause of their pain problem, or that the slightly abnormal vascular angiogram is the cause of their symptoms. Doing so can promote a lot of procedures that may or may not be necessary. A procedure may be done because of the induction of the nocebo; you believe it'll work, and it does for a period of time. So the nocebo promotes the procedure. It's the reason given by the provider; you believe it through the placebo effect and get better for a while.

I see it all the time. For a great engineer or technician, but not an honest one, the placebo keeps him or her in business. After a few months the patient is often running to return, with a new set of symptoms and the merry-go-round starts all over again—the merry-go-round of mind-body illnesses. That's where the money is. There is not much money in holistic teaching; I know, I do it every day. That's just fine because I'm doing my job as a physician. Remember, physician means teacher. I give multiple lectures to my patients every day. They listen to my CDs, watch DVDs, and read books that are relevant to their illness. Believe me, there's no money in this, just a lot of bills, but it sure makes me feel good. Many patients feel better for a period of time after they have a procedure done because of the "I believe" factor. I see it all the time. Two to three months later, the patient is walking up and down the mind-body index and seeing another doctor, many times one of a different specialty, and the nocebo and placebo start over again.

Providers must understand mind-body medicine, holistic medicine, but this is not taught in medical school. Recently, I had a chiropractic student making rounds for me at the hospital for a few days and I could not believe he knew nothing of mind-body medicine. He knew basic science very well, but didn't realize the brain was attached to the body. One would think that would be natural for a chiropractic student, but it was not. I know quite a few chiropractors that practice mind-body medicine, I'm happy to say. Frequently, they invite me to give lectures to their associations, and I appreciate that. The human body and mind give us false signals. At least 70 percent of the time chronic pain is a reflection of anxiety, stress, fear, and depression. It's just plainly a fraud. Chronic pain doesn't kill anybody and should not be the plague that it is to many people. So remember, "nocebo" doctors are extremely common and you must be aware of this. They may be excellent in their technique and get away with a lot of stuff because they're good at it, but the necessity of it is another matter altogether.

# Rudy's Holistic Pain Clinic

It's one thing to criticize the majority of today's pain clinics, but another to recommend a better one. The reason for starting a holistic pain clinic is to get away from all these procedures and addicting medications and make the patient well with less risk and cost. I don't think it would be easy to open a holistic freestanding pain clinic. I doubt a surgical group would ever do such a thing. I doubt hospitals would support it financially. I have one in a hospital, but I'm the owner of it. They could not make money off it; they get paid for procedures, that's where the money is. The majority of patients with severe chronic pain have no money, many are addicts, and a number are physically or psychologically disabled.

My mind-body institute is working fairly well because it is in a hospital and its main focus is wellness, not just pain. I'm developing a holistic pain clinic within it. I already have available a lot of the wellness modalities like massage, yoga, tai chi, mindfulness, personal training, weight reduction, Zumba dancing, etc.

The director of a pain clinic must have a thorough understanding of wellness and pain, and money cannot be at the top of this list. The pain centers today that do a lot of procedures certainly are where the money is. I could care less, and even congratulate them if they are getting people well with these procedures, but in my experience that is not the case the majority of the time. Yet, a holistic approach can provide a good living for many people and get a lot of people well. There is no doubt that the big cars, and the big houses, are not owned by the staff of the holistic pain centers. The spine surgeons and pain doctors own them, and we all know that. Then again, holistic medicine is starting to slowly spread across the country. There are currently many holistic pain centers in San Francisco and several in Canada.

Dr. Jon Kabat-Zinn was able to start a huge clinic outside Boston, so it can be done. His work on holistic pain is internationally known. Patients entering a holistic pain center should be given a long questionnaire to fill out regarding the history of their pain. I would also give them a yellow pad and a pencil and encourage them to write their story—the longer the better. The opening question of the provider should be, "What's going on in your life?" Not, "What is your pain?" There are many modalities that could be available in the pain clinic, but I suggest having ten to twenty and just being good at those.

As a provider, I would advertise in the newspapers and on TV, make some CDs and DVDs, and write books to give to patients, or suggest well-known pain books. Unfortunately, it is difficult to find holistic pain books. I've written one, *The Fraud of Chronic Pain*. I would also recommend Dr. Jon Kabat-Zinn's book also. I recommend giving lectures on the subject frequently and providing brochures for the referring doctors, especially psychiatrists.

You need to have a Web site that can be accessed easily, and pass out information, maybe even e-mail your patients. I send people to doctor's offices with brochures, make CDs and DVDs, and write books in order to educate the patient, the public, and fellow doctors.

A non-iconic approach is not an easy road, but it's the correct approach most of the time. Nobody dies from a holistic approach applied correctly to chronic pain. I think a mindful meditation class needs to be the center of every holistic approach. That's critical. In my book noted above I have an excellent chapter on mindfulness. It's a wonderful tool to teach stress reduction, pain reduction, etc.

Holistic, mindful medicine is the future. At first they will ignore us, then they will attack us, and then they will say they knew it all along. I heard former CEO John Mackey say that about the Whole Foods Market stores, and I think it applies equally to holistic medicine. Incidentally, I am 100 percent convinced that John Mackey feels the same about what I'm doing. He sent me an e-mail saying that. If you can shop at those stores, you will live a long time.

# Don't Be a Statistic

When average stats are thrown at you, such as, "Most are dead in six months," don't fall for them! There are always exceptions. Who knows for sure? Be exceptional.

Statistics also have a long curve or tail that can extend along through time, and some escape this statistic altogether. You never know where you are on the curve. In the domain of medical and radiation oncology, the mind aspect of healing is not even considered and is not in the statistics at all—a big mistake. New discoveries and methods of treatment are made daily and your odds could change in a second, so to throw in the towel is just plain ridiculous.

A change in treatment will change the median survival time and have a longer tail, and you might just live to a ripe old age.

# Statistics: Information, Not Condemnation

The objective, when you have cancer, is to find yourself in the long tail of the curve of the graph. No one can predict the course cancer will follow. Cancer is a puzzling business involving unpredictability and miracles. Take Lance Armstrong; he had multiple metastatics to the brain, but look at all the international races he won after that. Good medical treatment and positive thinking went a long way. Some patients who had numerous metastatics in the brain are alive a decade later. Why that is, no one knows for sure. It's probably the army, navy, and marines of your immunity. The link between resistance and disease progression, even from a purely ontological point of view, is still hard to tease apart. We have all heard of miracle cures, people who had only a few months to live and now are cured, or live for decades or years. We believe the spontaneous cures are rare, but maybe it's more common than we think. More escape the scientific studies because people gave up on them. Generally, the spontaneous cures are not in the stats.

At the Commonwealth Hospital in Southern California, patients try to take charge of their cancer, to learn to live in greater harmony with their bodies and to seek peace of mind. Using yoga, meditation, imaging, visualization techniques, and eating a proper diet, patients learn to live and fight the cancer, while avoiding those things that promote its development. Case histories show that this way they live two or three times longer than the average person with the same cancer at the same stage of development. *Dr. David Servan*-Schreiber] an oncologist from Pittsburgh objected to the statistics and said they are a select group that is just better educated, more motivated, and in better health. His view is mistaken, according to *Dr. David Servan*-Schreiber]; statistics showed that they beat the odds. It's very hard to establish double-blind studies; no two cases are alike, and the human mind cannot be duplicated or controlled. Indeed, those who are better informed about the disease, who look after the body and mind, and who are given what they need to improve their health, can mobilize their bodies with vital food to fight the cancer. Dr. Dean Ornish ran a double-blind study proving the value of diet, exercise, meditation, and yoga. All showed a dramatic response by the patients who practiced these versus people who did not follow his program. Also, the patients who followed his program had immune cells seven times more able to fight the cancer. The immune cells were more active against it. You can put statistics in their proper perspective and aim for a long tail at the right of the curve.

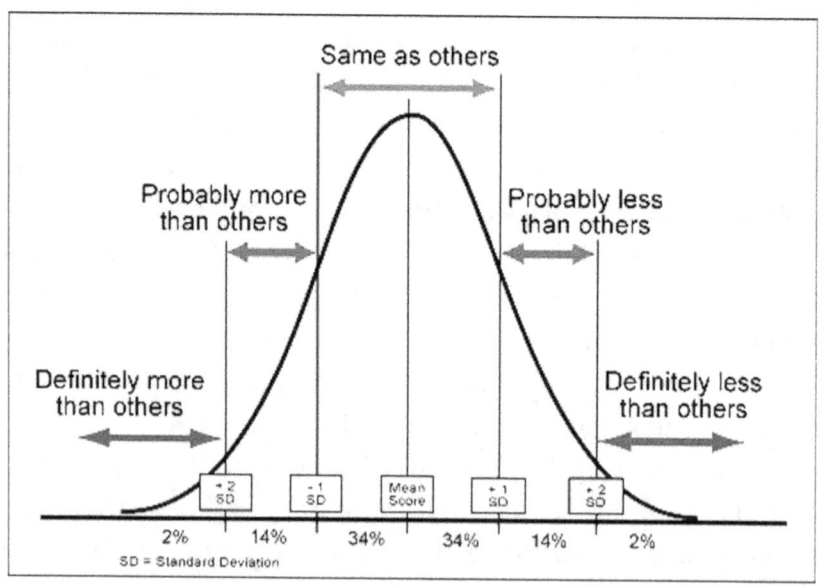

# The Body Has Multiple Brains

The heart has neuro cells in it, activated by the autonomic nervous system, the sympathetic and parasympathetic nervous system. We think, and the bowel reacts. This is done through somatic nerves, autonomic neurotransmitters, hormones, and neuropeptides. The heart has forty thousand neural cells, somatic nerves, sympathetic and parasympathetic. It is also affected by neuropeptides, hormones, and neurotransmitters. You can see that how we think is everything. It's a "heart-brain." The gastrointestinal tract has four hundred thousand neuro cells in it. Dr. Michael Gershon wrote a famous book, *The Second Brain*. The brain itself is one hundred billion neurons, and one hundred trillion neurotransmitters. Dr. Candace Pert details the connection of the mind and the body in her famous *Molecules of Emotion*, published in 1972, a great book to read. The skin is the largest organ in the body, covered by receptors on every cell. It has memory from all the neuropeptides, neurotransmitters, and hormones stimulating them. Yes, the skin has a brain.

## Heading for the Healing

Who are the survivors? Do they have certain personal attitudes? Psychologist Dr. Al Siebert studied the subject. One of the prominent characteristics was a fusion of opposites: serious and playful, tough and gentle, etc. Survivors have a hierarchy of needs and pursue all of them. The needs are self-esteem, self-actualization, and acceptance by others. The need for synergy is a big one. Survivors act from self-interest, but also from the interest of others.

Survivors characteristics:

- *Careers they like*
- *Remain at work and retire to work*
- *Receptive and creative*
- *High-end self-love and self-esteem*
- *Rarely docile*
- *Intelligent, with a strong sense of reality*
- *Concerned with others*
- *Don't lapse into depression*
- *Interpret problems as redirection*
- *Pessimism is a luxury they can't afford*

A new marriage, relationship, or job fulfilling a purpose in life are all common in the survivor history. Divorce, death, and loss of a job are common in the cancer industry. Dr. Siebert found that the survivor personality can be learned. Dr. Siebert lists the following indicators of self-motivated growth.

- *Aimless playfulness for its own sake, like that of a happy child.*
- *The ability to become so deeply absorbed in an activity that you lose track of time, external events, and all your worries.*
- *Humming, or talking to yourself absentmindedly.*
- *An innocent, childlike curiosity.*
- *An observant, nonjudgmental style.*
- *Willingness to look foolish, make mistakes, and laugh at yourself.*
- *Open-minded acceptance of criticism about yourself.*
- *An active imagination, daydreams, mental play, and conversations with yourself.*

Self-esteem, self-respect, and creativity are critical in the healing process. Emotional honesty and self-acceptance lead to better health. Becoming your own person releases your creativity. Freeing yourself from convention and what others might think is important.

To become the exceptional cancer patient that doubles his or her lifespan and increases his or her spontaneous and miraculous cure rate, you need to become a positive thinker. The works of Dr. Norman Vincent Peale are good to read: *You Can If You Think You Can*, *The Power of Positive Thinking*, and *Positive Imaging*. What you think about yourself is important. You must find a purpose in life that fits you and then live it. You're acting days are over and your profession is "being." Emotional honesty and self-acceptance lead to better physical health. Your brain is documenting this daily.

Women have better survival rates than men with the same cancer. Women are more accepting of their emotions. Men's emotions are around their work. Most cancer group therapy is composed of women. Psychologists estimate less than 20 percent of the population has a focus of control, the kind of self-passion in which persons are guided by their own standards and their beliefs about what others think. This integrity is a large part of the survivor personality. Development of individuality is a safeguard to life and health. This is found in rural areas more commonly because there, self-reliance is the standard. You release your own creativity when you become self-reliant. Then, you are your own person. The mind bonds with new solutions, new goals, and creativity, and the healing begins. As Dr. Hans Seelye, the famous stress researcher, said, "If you do what you like, you never really work, your work is your play." This only works if you are someplace you would rather be. If we become survivors, we realize a deeper need to love and be at peace, and motivation becomes selfless, not selfish. The knowledge that when we die we have given something to the world is important. In the process, we create a sense of worth that helps us achieve goals that improve the quality of our lives and those of others.

Visualization and meditation can accomplish the transformation quickly. Imaging channels mental energy toward the desired result, and acting on it brings the desired results.

Don't be a statistic. Make a plan and be exceptional. None of us can predict tomorrow—cancer or no cancer, life or death. Don't get stuck in a time frame. Try to set realistic targets that are achievable with confidence and self-worth. Look at the future with optimism. "He who has a why to live can bear almost any how" (Nietzsche). The goal is to live for yourself in a selfless way that also helps others. Again, meditation and visualization are powerful tools and send messages to the subconscious mind to achieve your goals. You create hope in giving a "live" message. Our thought process affects seventy trillion body cells, positively or negatively. How you think is everything.

Ten years ago, I saw a patient with a malignant primary brain tumor. After telling him what it was all about, with at best a few months to a year or two to live, I gave him an exaggerated 10 percent chance of survival. He said, in no uncertain terms, "I'm not going to die!" I said immediately, "I will do everything I can to help you," and we gave each other a hug. He lived up to his promise to follow everything scientifically possible and I constantly worked on his power of positive thinking. He lived eight years with a horrible malignancy. When he died, his CT scan the week before had shown only brain atrophy—no evidence of the tumor. It seemed to me that he just got tired of living, and I had noticed a change in his attitude. We had a very cooperative partnership.

Dr. Bernie Siegel has some recommendations for your hospital stay, if one is necessary.

- *Dress as an individual—the heck with hospital clothes!*
- *Decorate the room with family and spirituality; demand a room with a window.*
- *Know why they are running those tests on you.*
- *Have books, CDs, DVDs, and music in your room (I even provide a CD and DVD player for the patient if he wishes to use it).*
- *Have them play CDs during your surgery.*
- *Speak to your own body—your neurotransmitters*
- *Pray with your family, spiritual leader, and even your doctor*

So far we have discussed some psychological predispositions for cancer and how to possibly avoid them in order to increase your lifespan and your chances of a spontaneous cure. We will teach you how to relax through meditation and breathing techniques, and then teach you imaging and visualization methods of attacking the cancer itself. These have been well described in other books, and references will be made throughout the book and found at the end for further reading. I will teach you how to use mental techniques to decrease stress and stimulate your immune system—your army, navy, and air force—to work for you. Patients mistrust their body and its ability to destroy disease. Learning to relax through meditation will help you to accept and use your body to become well again. Stress increases fear and relaxation helps to decrease it. Fear can become overwhelming when people are faced with a life-threatening disease. Cancer patients are often terrified that they will die a long, painful death and destroy their family economically in the process. Such fears make it difficult to develop a positive life expectancy. Patients develop a different perception when using relaxation techniques. Exercise is a way of lowering stress; I do it regularly and it works for me. Exercise activates endorphins, our body's morphine, and decreases or eliminates our fight-or-flight response.

Dr. Herbert Benson of Harvard writes a lot about relaxation and meditation techniques in his book *The Relaxation Response*. Dharma Singh Khalsa, MD, also writes about other relaxation techniques in his famous book *Meditation As Medicine*. Now, let's get down to specifics.

# Progressive Relaxation

Dr. Edmund Jacobson invented a program called Progressive Relaxation. I've made a few additions to it from my own experience.

1. *Pick a spiritual place—home, office, church, or whatever is convenient for daily use.*
2. *Use soft lighting. Close the door. Sit in a chair or lie down on the floor.*

3. *Pay attention to your breathing, starting with the nose. It will center your mind. Think of nothing else.*
4. *Take deep diaphragmatic breaths like a baby. Relax the belly.*
5. *Relax all your muscles, your whole body, starting with your face.*
6. *Visualize the relaxation. Take about ten to twenty deep breaths.*
7. *Use a mantra, fixating on a word or image if you cannot quiet your mind.*
8. *This should take about five minutes.*

## Moving Into Mental Imagery

The mind has an unbelievable capacity for mental imaging, even memory experts or technicians will testify to that. Look at a visual image; you will not forget it. Continue to picture yourself in a very relaxed state for two or three minutes; then, mentally picture the cancer in either realistic or symbolic terms. Think of the cancer as consisting of very weak, confused cells. Remember that our bodies destroy cancer cells thousands of times during a normal lifetime, probably daily. As you picture your cancer, realize that your recovery requires your body's own defenses and return to a natural, healthy state. Form a great visualization of your army, navy, and air force that are working for you. Picture your treatment coming into your body in a way that you understand. If you are receiving radiation treatment, picture it as a beam of millions of bullets of energy killing the cancer cells in their path. The normal cells are able to repair any damage that is done, but the cancer cells cannot because they're weak. If you are receiving chemotherapy, picture a drug coming into your body and entering the bloodstream. Picture the drug acting like a poison. The normal cells are intelligent and strong and don't take up the poison so readily. But the cancer cell is a weak cell and it takes very little to kill it. It absorbs the poison, dies, and is flushed out of your body. Picture your body's own white cells coming into the area where the cancer is, recognizing the abnormal cells, and destroying them. There is a vast army of white cells. They are very strong and aggressive. They are also very smart. There is no contest between them and the cancer cells, and they will win the battle. Picture the cancer shrinking. See the dead cells being carried away by the white cells, flushed from your body through the liver and kidneys, and eliminated in the urine and stool. Visualize some color to it; the wilder the visualization, the better. Remember, visualizations have great power in the human mind. Continue to see the cancer shrinking until it is all gone. If you are experiencing pain anywhere in your body, picture the army of white cells flowing into that area and soothing the pain. Visualize your body becoming well. Picture yourself reaching your goals in life; see your purpose in life being fulfilled, the members of your family doing well, and your relationships with people around you becoming more meaningful. Remember that having strong reasons for being well will help get you well, so use this time to focus clearly on your priorities in life. Give yourself a mental pat on the back for participating in the recovery. Do this mental imagery exercise three times per day, about fifteen minutes per session, staying awake and alert as you do it. Let the muscles in your eyelids lighten up, get ready to open your eyes, and become aware of the room and ready to resume your usual activities.

Take time now to go through this mental image of the process and practice it a few times.

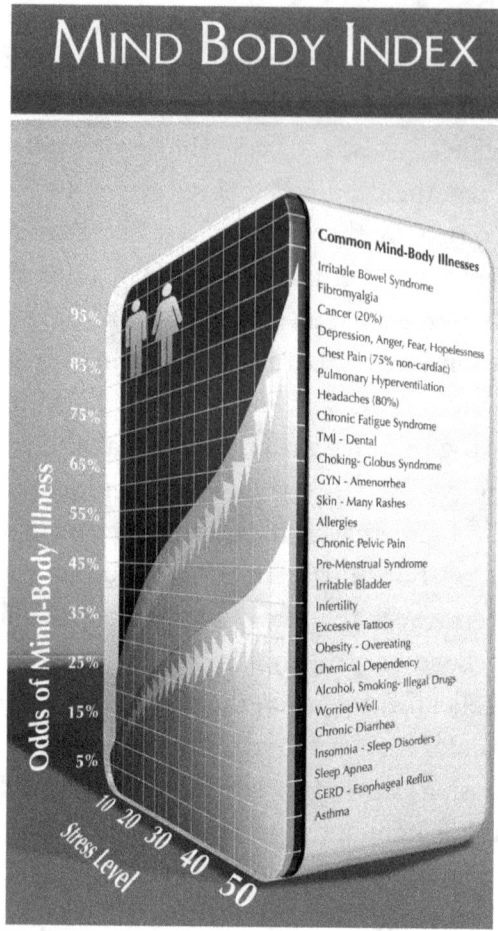

## The Mind-Body Index and Mental Imagery

The mental imaging process can be used for any of the illnesses on my mind-body index, or frankly any illness or disease. The mind is part of every human condition and can be used for healing. For example, it could be used for any pain problem: headaches, fibromyalgia, irritable bowel, skin rashes, etc. Create a mental picture of any ailment or pain that you have now. Visualize it in a form that makes sense to you. Picture any treatment you're receiving and see it eliminating the source of the ailment or pain and strengthening your body's ability to heal itself.

Imagine yourself healthy and free of the ailment or pain. See yourself proceeding successfully to meeting your goals in life.

# Spirituality and Healing

I commonly pray with my patient both before and after surgery. I learned that from a famous neurosurgeon, Dr. John Tew, from Cincinnati, who said, "It works and patients do better!" Dr. Bernie Siegel said, "Render unto the surgeon, radiation therapists, and medical oncologist to do what they can according to their ability and unto God what is his." I truly believe all need to work together, and I have seen the results. Patient, doctor, and spirituality need to work in unison. Dr. Siegel believes the following are crucial for recovery from serious illness, and I totally agree.

- *Faith in oneself*
- *Faith in one's doctor*
- *Faith in one's treatment*
- *One's spiritual faith*

Spirituality or religion creates meaning or order in the universe. The force behind creation is a loving intellectual energy. Spirituality means acceptance of what is.

In other words, I believe in the sun even if it doesn't shine, I believe in love even when I'm not shown it, I believe in God even when he does not speak. Spirituality means the ability to find peace and happiness in an imperfect world. Acceptance, faith, forgiveness, peace, and love are traits that define spirituality. These characteristics are traits Dr. Siegel always found in those who achieved unexpected healing of a serious illness—persons who believed in the benevolent higher power as a potent reason for hope. It's hard to find peace in life if you believe death is a meaningless end of an earthly existence. Life is not futile. We need to take advantage of what is in our own belief system, which is different for all of us.

A man with cancer is told by his primary physician that he will be dead in an hour. He runs to the window, looks up at the sky and says, "God, save me!" Out of the blue comes a wonderful, melodious voice, saying, "Don't worry, my son. I will save you!" The man climbs back into bed feeling reassured. His physician calls him a few hours later and says, "If I operate on you within an hour, I can save you." The man says, "No thanks, God will save me!" Then the oncologist, the radiation thera-pist, and the nutritional therapist all tell him, "We can save you!" The patient replies, "I don't need you, God will save me!" In an hour the man dies. When he gets to heaven, he walks up to God and says, "What happened? You said you'd save me and here I am, dead!" And God says, "You dumbbell! A sensible surgeon, an oncologist, a radiation therapist, and a nutritional therapist told you they could save you, and you did not take advantage of the cure." In other words, we need to use all four faiths as recommended by Dr. Siegel.

# Ageless Living

Many people are not living their age anymore. Adults dress like young-sters and youngsters dress like adults. A health culture is practiced in their senior years by a good 10 to 20 percent of the community, espe-cially the more educated and economically better off. Some live in age-less housing communities where one must be fifty-five and over to enter. Cosmetic procedures are done and they all look alike. Age-appropriate behavior is going by the wayside. A significant number just keep on working. Some need to do that for economic reasons, due to no retire-ment planning; others, like me, just frankly love it. Some have their children when in their fifties. Hugh Hefner married a woman sixty years his junior.

Woody Allen never rests, directing one movie every year. "I just love it," he says. They ignore aging; have new goals, aspirations, and purpose; and age without getting old. By 2050, one-fifth of humans will be sixty-five and older. But the Hayflick limit is still at work; you can do only so much. Your body cells will stop dividing eventually.

Cenegenics is the study of aging, paving the road to a long life. Maybe even immortality, as Catherine Mayer would call it. Her book *Amortality: The Pleasures and Perils of Living Agelessly*, is a combination of nutrition, exercise, and hormone optimization.

I personally don't approve of hormone replacement because of serious unknown and potentially irreversible side effects. There are a lot of side effects with androgen therapy. Underpinning the medications, sex hormones, and growth hormones is the notion that hormone replacement can return us to our natural state of youth. Testosterone can increase muscle mass, but also has a lot of other side effects. Decreased sperm production, increased cholesterol, decreased testicular size, bad skin, high fluid retention, and who knows what else. Again, I don't recommend it. Even increased rates of cancer are beginning to appear in the hormone replacement literature. Aging and staying young is a state of mind that defies measurement but can be greatly influenced by following the principle of the longevity mind-body index (www.kachmannmindbody.com).

# Intimacy, Love, and Healing

I have always admired and appreciated the books and scientific articles of Dr. Dean Ornish, one of the first holistic healers. He has published literature about healthy eating, and the prevention, stopping, and reversing of vascular disease. Also, he's always looked at the benefits of exercise and the psychological aspect of healing. It is my opinion that what he recommends for vascular disease works just as well for the prevention and treatment of many aspects of cancer. His book *Love and Survival* would apply to all medical illnesses and diseases.

I have a friend at the lake named Max who was told fifteen years ago that he needed a heart transplant. I gave him the books and DVDs of Dr. Dean Ornish, and he's alive and well at age seventy-five, building houses in Marion, Indiana. He follows the recommendations of Dr. Ornish closely. I recommend and teach this in my books. Dr. Ornish pays particular attention to the mind aspect of healing. He considers close relationships, family, community, intimacy, and love to be of great benefit to health.

His published scientific papers state that 80 percent of the patients who were eligible for coronary heart bypass surgery and followed his programs safely avoided surgery by making comprehensive lifestyle changes.

The combination of diet, love, and intimacy affect a multitude of diseases, including cancer. Our survival depends on the healing power of love, intimacy, and relationships. It plays a huge part. The healing power of emotion and spiritual transformation can be as powerful as the diet or surgery.

Dr. Ornish feels that today's focus is primarily on the physical, mechanistic, drugs, and surgery.

## Not Everything That Counts Can Be Counted

Many physicians, especially me, are finding that practicing medicine only as a mechanic, technician, plumber, or engineer does not feed their soul, and it is leaving their patients without proper treatment and little hope. The only side effects of changing one's attitude or diet are good ones. Reducing prostate cancer, breast cancer, colon cancer, lymphoma, diabetes, arthritis, and obesity can all be done by switching to a high-nutrient-dense way of eating. The true physician is more than just a plumber, technician, or mechanic. I recently asked the person in charge of the third- and fourth-year students at the IU–Purdue medical school if I could give some lectures on holistic healing. The woman said they had no time for that. This upset me somewhat, and I said, "You should be handing out engineering degrees to the med school class from Purdue. You are not graduating doctors." Incidentally, we are still friends; I was just passing on my forty-two years of experience. We all have an emotional heart, a psychological heart, and a spiritual heart. Our heart has forty thousand neural cells; our bowels have four hundred thousand. So how we think has a great effect on the heart, bowels, and immunity to fight cancer.

## Loneliness and Isolation Promote Disease

Pain is a message, that it's time for a change. Fifty to 70 percent of pain is psychologically based. Real pain and suffering are not the same. Suffering is more common. Curing is wonderful, but healing takes you away from the suffering and is more difficult to achieve. Viktor Frankl's famous book based on his concentration camp experience, *Man's Search for Meaning*, is very interesting to read. He found if you establish control, congruity, and commitment it greatly increases your chances of surviving a horrible situation like that of a Nazi death camp or serious illness. Many of the cancer survivors and treating physicians have mentioned that to me. The sense of meaning was different for many. Sometimes suffering of any kind gets your attention. We read how important relationships, love, and intimacy are, and researchers found that the number and quality of relationships are important. How numerous and loving are your support groups? Social support is defined as information leading the subject to believe that he is cared for and loved, that he has a network in place and is mutually supportive. It is the experience and perception of loving relationships that seem to determine their effect on our health. Perception is reality. Community means people in the neighborhood.

# What's Love Got to Do with It?

The idea that social support can affect disease is contrary to Koch's postulates. He discovered bacteria, the first infectious agent to be discovered. His friend Pasteur, who developed the germ theory, said on his deathbed, "The microbe is nothing, the soil is everything." Dr. Dean Ornish quoted numerous large studies in his book *Love and Survival* to support the benefits of intimacy, love, and healing. I will review just one of them: the Rosetta Study. One of the earliest and most important studies recognizing the power of love and relationships to modify the harmful effects of otherwise unhealthy behaviors was conducted in Rosetta, an Italian American town in eastern Pennsylvania. Rosetta has been studied intensively for over fifty years.

The population of Rosetta was found to have a strikingly low mortality rate from heart attacks and other illnesses, including cancer. During the first thirty years, it was studied and compared to Bangor, an immediately adjacent town, and Nazareth, a neighboring town. The same hospital facilities, water supply, and physicians served all three communities. Why was the incidence of heart attacks and other illnesses so much lower in Rosetta? Rosetta had been settled in 1882 by immigrants from a town in southern Italy, and they still displayed a high level of ethnic and social homogeneity, close family ties, and cohesive community relationships. They were right. In the late 1960s and 1970s, there was a shift from households with strong commitments to religion, relationships, and traditional values and practices to a less cohesive, fragmented, and isolated community. This loosening of family ties and weakening of the community in Rosetta was accompanied by a substantial increase in deaths due to heart attacks and other illnesses, including cancer. The China study, a clinic study of one billion Chinese people, also proved that what you eat and life-style had a great effect on the rate of vascular disease and cancer. Numerous other studies have proved that. Medical school doesn't teach the value of love and intimacy. Group support has been proven to be especially helpful to patients with metastatic breast cancer. It also has been shown that women are much more responsive to mind-body techniques and healing, especially love and intimacy. It has been my experience, from my Mind-Body Spirit Center I have at Lutheran Hospital, that women are a lot more intuitive and more in touch with their emotions. So my teaching has more value to them. Most of the people in our classes and attending my lectures on mind-body medicine are female. Men tend to give up, especially single men. Men's emotions are much more tied to their work. I was talking over lunch one day to a friend of mine, a radiation oncologist, and he said, "Especially single young men, when diagnosed with cancer, die very quickly, versus married men or women." Another psychological factor that has a profound influence on premature death and disease is hostility. Those who scored in the upper 20 percent of hostility when tested twenty years earlier had a 42 percent increased risk of premature death from all causes combined, including heart disease and cancer, when compared to those who scored in the lower 20 percent of hostility. The effects of hostility are equal to or are greater in magnitude than the traditional risk factors for heart disease: elevated cholesterol, high blood pressure, etc. Dealing with the underlying loneliness can be healing. Commitment leads to trust, intimacy, and healing. Fear leads to no commitment, mistrust, cynicism, hostility, isolation, disease, and premature death. Your immune system is less effective when you're in conflict with your spouse or companion, even when you are newly married and are otherwise happy. Instead, be a spouse of refuge, love, and support. It's potentially distressing when your spouse is a source of conflict. Women are more likely to show negative immunological changes than are men. Remember, women are more in touch with their emotions. Dr. Ornish would say, "Open your heart for healing with good family and social support." Intimacy is liberating and healing, but only if you feel safe. Opening your heart is just another way of saying that you're willing to let down your defenses and allow yourself to be emotionally vulnerable.

# The Road to Love and Healing

The path to intimacy, love, and increased immunity is on my mind-map. There are multiple ways, roads, intersections, and opportunities. It's not a straight path like a normal love relationship most of the time. So pick a path with a heart and open your heart, as Dr. Dean Ornish would say. It is important to start with awareness of your mind-body connection. My book *Welcome to Your Mind Body* tells you the physiology of the effects of the mind on the body and body on the mind. If you make a commitment to the journey of healing, you will need to listen to CDs, watch DVDs, and become motivated to participate in the process. You will see that doors will open for you. "Ask and it will be given to you; seek and you will find; knock and the door will open unto you." Spiritual practice is what you are thinking. You have a choice to keep your heart open or closed to love or fear. The willingness to feel vulnerable and open your heart is essential to real intimacy. Communication is a fundamental skill for building positivity, contact, commitment, and community. Hearing thoughts as judgment and criticism closes a heart. We tend to look at feelings in a different way, with an open heart.

Feeling are so true. Thoughts can be argued about. Thoughts keep us stuck in the past. Emotions influence us more than thoughts. Advertisements, political and fund-raising campaigns, and propaganda have more illogical thoughts than facts. The ability to feel another's emotions is a path to compassion.

The road to healing, love, and intimacy:

1. *Identify what you feel.*
2. *Disclose what you feel.*
3. *Listen carefully to what another person is feeling.*
4. *Acknowledge the other person's feelings and empathize with care and compassion.*

# Group Therapy

Group therapy provides a safe place for people to consciously let down their emotional defenses and barriers in order to experience and express their emotions and be open to healing each other. When people open their hearts to each other healing often happens. As we well know, women are much more into the mind aspect of healing, and group therapy is effective for breast cancer as well as for other mind-body illnesses. There are many types of support group therapies available. Part of what makes support groups so powerful is that people feel they are not alone. A support group provides an environment where real feelings and emotions can be expressed. "What's really going on in my life?" Identify what you're feeling, disclose what you're feeling, listen carefully to what another person is feeling, and acknowledge the other person by feeling with empathetic care and compassion. Commitment, touch, and meditation are powerful tools to open your heart, and they lead to intimacy, love, and healing.

# Visualization and Imagery – The Road to Healing

The healing power of visualization and imagery in the brain is huge.

We all know that the greatest athletes use visualization to perfect their performance. The greatest golfers in the world are of the greatest visualizers. When they step up to hit the ball they're visualizing the shot. When I step up to serve in tennis, I visualize a complete shot before I hit it. I've been doing that for years. Until I started writing a book on memory and doing a lot of research, I did not realize that the greatest memoirists use imaging and visualization and connect it to a number, word, or object. They use wild and imaginative images and the power of their memory is unbelievable. What it's really telling us is that the brain has a fantastic imaging power. I knew it was there, but I did not realize the extent of it. We need to take full advantage of it. I'm going to explain to you, in detail, the power of it and how it works. Visualization is the language of the unconscious mind. As already mentioned, the best sports pros generally are the best visualizers. Just ask Arnold Palmer or Tiger Woods. Whether you recover from cancer depends on many factors, of course: the type of tumor, its stage, its aggressiveness, its location, the effectiveness of the treatment, your general health, what you eat, whom you are treated by, and most importantly, what you are willing to participate in for the healing. The purpose of using your mind is to increase the likelihood that you will have the outcome you want. According to Martin L. Rossman, MD, the benefits of imaging are:

1. *Imagery is comforting and tremendously stress relieving.*
2. *Imagery stimulates your immune system.*
3. *Imagery is enjoyable.*
4. *Imagery is better than worrying.*
5. *Imagery can relieve pain.*
6. *Imagery can prevent or reduce the nausea from chemotherapy drugs.*
7. *Imagery can prevent complications and pain after surgery.*
8. *Imagery can reduce stress during radiation therapy.*
9. *Imagery can expand your awareness of your body, feelings, mind, and spirit.*
10. *Imagery can help you access strength and courage.*
11. *Imagery can connect you to your creativity and problem-solving abilities.*
12. *Imagery can enhance your intuitive abilities and help with decision making.*
13. *Imagery can help you connect with your own spirituality.*
14. *Imagery can help you find peace of mind.*

# What Is Imagery?

Imagery consists of thoughts that can be seen, heard, smelled, tasted, or sensed in some way in your mind. Memories, dreams, fantasies, plans, illusions, and lies all involve imagery. Art involves imagery; it's the language of poetry, painting, music, myths, and dreams. Imagery is a way of thinking. You can use it to relax, fight cancer, relieve pain, and increase immunity. It is used to generate creativity and to process and manage emotions. As we may already know, the first skill in imaging is to learn how to relax. In other words, get into a meditative mood.

Imagery stimulates your creativity and helps find solutions to difficult problems, like cancer. It can be used to increase courage, patience, tolerance, humor, self-confidence, and support your cancer treatment. Imagery is a natural way of thinking, but few of us have been trained in it. Imagery can be thought of as major coding languages. An abstract system using words and numbers allows us to name and quantify things. The second coding system is imagery. It is the language or coding system utilized by a simultaneous information process; a mode of thinking which tends to perceive how things are related as a part of the bigger whole. It lets us look at the tapestry into which things are woven. It helps us grasp the bigger picture. Like a painting, it may not be logical, but still it is very meaningful and makes its own kind of emotional sense. Imagery is clearly tied to our emotions; it is not sequential like numbers and words.

Emotions are important in mind-body healing. They motivate us to action, and also produce physiological changes in the body through hormones, neurotransmitters, and neuropeptides. Modern research in psycho-neural-immunology (PNI) points to the emotions as the key modulator of chemical secretions by the brain, gut, and immune system. The body tends to respond to imaging as it would to genuine external experience. Imaging has been shown in numerous research studies to affect almost all major physiological control systems of the body, including breathing, heart, blood pressure, metabolic states, G.I. function, sexual function, and an immune response. With guided imagery, the coding language of the mind influences physiology, stimulates healing, creates relaxation, and connects us with wisdom and strength. When the immune system is stimulated by imagery, there are no adverse side effects. Any side effects actually tend to be positive, with a greater sense of empowerment and feelings of wholeness.

## Let's Cut to the Chase

Your immune cells—your T cells—are the army, navy, and air force that will save your life. All of us develop a few abnormal cells every day and our immune cells immediately destroy them. So there is a great need to mobilize our defenses when we have cancer. It has been proven that how we think can affect our immune cell activity. Our thymus gland is the biggest source of our T cells. So the use of visual and guided imaging techniques to mobilize them would be natural. Dr. Belleruth Naparstek, in her book *Staying Well with Guided Imagery*, describes a great immune cell imagery.

## Immune Cell Imagery

Start by making yourself comfortable, shifting your weight so you feel supported, whether you are sitting or lying down. Try to see to it that your head, neck, and spine are straight. Let your eyes close. Take a deep, cleansing breath, inhaling as fully as you comfortably can. Take another breath, deep into the belly, and breathe out as fully as possible. Once more, breathe in and imagine that you're sending the energy of your breath to any part of your body that is sore or tense, releasing the tension with the exhale. Feel your breath going to all the tight, tense places and softening them. Gather up all the tension and breathe it out so that more and more you feel safe and comfortable, relaxed and at ease. Watch the cleansing action of the breath with a friendly and detached awareness. Any unwelcome thoughts that come to mind can be sent out with the breath, with a friendly but detached awareness. For just a moment, the mind is empty; it is free and clear and you are blessed with stillness. The emotional self can be still and quiet, like a lake with no ripples. Now, put the palm of one hand over your breastbone, a little below the base of your neck. Put your other hand on the center of your belly, also palm down. Feel the healing warmth that is coming out of your hands and softly entering your body, gently penetrating into skin, muscle, and bone, layer by layer, surrounding and soaking into the glands. That's how your immune cells stimulate and revitalize them. Perhaps even feel a ripple of fresh appreciation for the constant support and protection they provide. Feel the thymus (the master T cell gland), somewhere beneath your hand, gearing up to send forth whatever armies of immune cells are needed to any place in the body to eliminate anything that might harm you. Loyal and ready, there are thousands of miraculous little soldier cells; highly trained, focused, intelligent, and totally committed to your well-being, knowing what to attack and what to leave alone—your army, navy, and air force. These highly trained fighter cells can immediately see the cancer cell has made itself at home; the telltale damaged DNA readily identifies the abnormal cell like muddy footprints at the entrance of a house. Sense the patrolling T cells as they sight the cancer cells, quickly surrounding and destroying them with a deft thrust like a fall in the hands of a master fencer, shutting them down forever. Know that these miraculous little T cells can even clone themselves if necessary, and can spread out in multiples of themselves after other cancer cells, ferociously pursuing each and every one with commitment, focus, and determination. Healthy cells survey the action and call in more troops as needed, and suppressor cells that are able to see when the last of the enemy is gone. So feel peaceful and easy; you are on the road to healing.

# Emotional Resilience

When we are told that we have a life-threatening illness like cancer, understandably we feel threatened. So our resiliency to help ourselves will be tested. Imagery that is specifically geared to help with physical symptoms and body elements will automatically help with mood and emotion at the same time. Great images help with emotions. Foster a relaxed appreciation of self and provide a kind of protective "emotional cushion" that slows down the psychic wear and tear of daily living. This is true when you are listening to imagery that helps the body to eliminate cancer cells and helps the psyche rinse stress and relieve grief. First we need to be able to acknowledge and tolerate our own feelings, whatever they are. This keeps us in touch with ourselves, supplements us with vital data for our own health and safety, and allows us to release the emotions we would otherwise be holding. Second, we need to feel safe, but maintain the protection of strong, healthy boundaries. Otherwise, we aren't able to protect ourselves from others and run the risk of violating them. This is the interpersonal component. Thirdly, we need to increase our general self-esteem by understanding and appreciating who we really are and what we have to give to the world. With self-esteem comes the motivation and empowerment to express who we are and what we have to give. Ultimately, self-esteem is about connecting fully to a sense of purpose and our life's meaning, so this component is about our relationship to the world at large.

# Faith and Healing

Dr. Norman Vincent Peale preached his ministry in New York City at the Marble Church and all over the world. He tried to connect the spiritual mind living in your physical mind and health. His famous books include *The Power of Positive Thinking, You Can If You Think You Can, Positive Imaging*, and about thirty other books, lectures, CDs, and DVDs.

Even a psychiatric institute is attached to his church in New York City. He knew the importance of the human mind, spirituality, and faith, and connected it to stress reduction, decreased depression, and healing; and created a better world for thousands of people, maybe even millions.

Three years ago, I operated on the girlfriend of an eighty-eight-year-old minister who worked for Dr. Peale. He noticed the many newspaper articles written about me which decorate the wall of my office (to keep the patients busy while they're waiting for me, and also to get to know me a bit better; I want them to know I'm a holistic doctor in spite of being a surgeon). The girlfriend had had a good result from the operation I performed on her, and the minister showed his appreciation by giving me twenty-one of Dr. Peale's books, autographed by him and his wife, Ruth. To me, a real treasure trove. (From them, I made six hundred PowerPoint slides for lectures, which are on my Web site, www.kachmannmindbody.com). I had forgotten the name of the patient. I wanted him to give the opening prayer in my lecture on the power of positive thinking. On a Sunday night before my lecture on Monday, guess who passes right by me at Parkview Hospital ICU? The minister that formerly worked for Dr. Peale and gave me all those books. What do you think? A God event? I certainly think so. He was at my lecture the following night.

The point is that Dr. Peale had a lifetime of experience with faith and healing. At first he was skeptical, not totally convinced that faith could affect healing. He says now that faith properly understood and applied is a powerful factor in overcoming disease and in the establishment of health. Many medical professionals agree with what he says, including me. I've been practicing forty-two years and am only thirty-nine years old—ha! Dr. Peale's attitude turned in the direction of faith and healing after he met a gentleman at one of his lectures, who told him the following story:

A number of years ago he had a malady that was diagnosed as osteoma of the jaw; that is, a bone tumor that is malignant. The doctor told him it was practically incurable. You can imagine how that disturbed him. Desperately he looked for help. Although he had attended church regularly, he was still not a particularly religious man. One day, however, as he lay in bed, it occurred to him that he would like to read the Bible. He asked his wife to bring one to him. She was very surprised, since he had never before made such a request. He began to read, and found consolation and comfort. He also became a bit more hopeful and less discouraged. He continued to read every day. But that wasn't the chief result. He began to notice that the condition which had troubled him was growing less noticeable. At first he thought he imagined this; then, he became convinced that some change was taking place in him. One day while reading the Bible, an inward feeling of warmth, great happiness, and appreciation developed. It was difficult to describe. From that time on his improvement was more rapid. He went to the doctors who first diagnosed the case. They were all surprised that his condition had improved, but warned him that it was only a temporary respite. Later, however, upon further examination, it was determined that the symptoms of osteoma had disappeared entirely. Still the doctors told him it would probably start all over again. This did not disturb him, for in his heart he knew that he was healed. How long had it been since the healing? Dr. Peale asked. "Fourteen years" was his answer.

There are many stories like that out there, a number of which I will relate later in a separate section. This growing emphasis on present-day religious practice, which is designed to help people find the healing from the sickness of mind, body, and soul, goes back to ancient times. Only recently have doctors become engineers, not healers, and in many instances it definitely is a problem. There are some holistic cancer centers, but many are not. It frankly is not taught in medical school. I know because I've experienced it almost daily. Many make the false assumption that science and religion don't mix. Spirituality means accepting the moment without judgment, that's all. So don't bring in the whole scientific community in dealing with spirituality. Both are needed. Now the association of religion and science is starting to be recognized in some places. Large religious organizations are starting to accept the theory of evolution. Science and religion can exist together. Remember, *holiness* is derived from the word *wholeness*.

Meditation closely resembles the root word of medicine. Since religion deals with thoughts and feelings and basic attitudes, it's only natural that the science of faith should be important in the healing process. There is empirical evidence to support the belief that God works in both the practitioners of science, the doctors, and the practitioners of faith, the ministers. How you think affects the neurotransmitters, hormones, neuropeptides, and T cells—the army, navy, and air force of your immunity. Dr. Peale received a letter from an upstate physician that noted 60 percent of patients were sick in their minds and souls—exactly my experience after forty-two years. It is hard to realize that the modern soul is sick to such an extent that it can cause illness. Seventy-five percent of the patients who see a doctor need only a good coach. A better understanding of our emotional selves and a return to religious faith seems to form the combination that holds the great promise of personal health for many of us.

Dr. Peale says that in the investigations of successful cases of healing, there seem to be certain factors present. First, a complete surrender of all of oneself into the hands of God. Second, completely letting go of all errors, such as sin in any form, and a desire to be cleansed in the soul. Thirdly, belief and faith in the combined therapy of medical science in harmony with the healing power of God. Fourth, a sincere willingness to accept God's answer, whatever it may be, with no irritability or bitterness against his will. Fifth, a substantial, unquestioning faith that God can help. And actually, in every case that Peale examined, in one form or another the patient talks about a moment when he was warm and full of beauty, peace, joy, and a sense of relief, leading to the healing.

Here are eight practical suggestions:

1. *In sickness, send for your religious leader and of course a good mix of health-care providers, such as your family doctor and oncologist.*

2. *Pray for the doctor. Realize that God uses trained humans to mentally aid in the healing process. Do not abandon scientific medical care professionals. After all, God sent them to you. "The doctor treats the patient and God heals him."*

3. *Don't pick up anything that would send negative thoughts and interfere with the healing.*

4. *Remember, you will heal through the natural laws of science, and the other things bring healing by spiritual laws applicable through faith.*

5. *Completely surrender yourself into the hands of God. By your faith you can place yourself in the flow of divine power. His healing is there, but in order to be effective, you must be completely released to God's will.*

6. *It is also important that harmony prevails in the family; that is, a spiritual harmony.*

7. *Form a picture in your mind of you being well. Imaging has great healing power.*

# You Can If You Think You Can

In my experience, cancer patients who double their life span or have an unexpected or miraculous healing all seem to have a similar way of thinking consistent with creativity, instead of a destructive mentality. Certainly, life-threatening problems can be overwhelming. But frankly, nothing in the world is certain. Never quit. Don't develop a defeatist psychology. Come at the problem from a different way. If the new approach fails to get you well, try another. For there is a key, there always is, a continual and thoughtful way. An undeviating search and attitude will produce it. Just think, don't get emotional, and hold to the basic principle that it is always too soon to quit. You'll usually get an idea if you think and don't panic. Never talk defeat. Don't say, "I can't do it!" Hayes Jones, a former Olympic runner, had a home for people like himself, who at one time felt defeated. It's the plugging away that will win you the day.

Just draw on your grip. It's so easy to quit. It's the keeping your chin up that's hard. It's easy for crawfish to crawl but difficult to fight when hope's out of sight. It's the living that's hard. The refusal to quit is called the persistence principle. It energizes you and then you will persevere. Keep at it and you'll get results. I don't accept a death sentence or deadlines. I don't accept the poor prognosis. If at first you don't succeed, try again. Your own perception is critical; you must perceive a positive thought stream and cultivate your own inner power. Don't be your own worst enemy. The hardest person to know is oneself. We hide from ourselves and don't face reality. It's inner conflict or mental conflict that defeats us. You must see yourself as you really are and deal with yourself honestly. Stand in front of a mirror and say, "I want the truth about you!" Every problem contains the seeds of its own solution. Problems are a sign of life. You only get strong if you have struggled. Don't bring me your success, it weakens me. Bring me your problems, they strengthen me.

# Anxiety and Fear

Anxiety, especially when caused by a life-threatening illness, is the "great modern plague." Panic won't do it. Almost any problem will yield to the "know-how and why" of knowledge and understanding. Thomas Edison said, "The only reason we need the body is to carry the brain around." The brain is dominant and that's why it's sitting on top. When a problem like cancer strikes, we react emotionally rather than think about it logically. The human mind will not function creatively when it is distressed. Hysteria keeps the surface of the mind in a state of disturbance. In addition to cool thinking, also make use of prayer.

Prayer is actually a line of communication along which comes insight, intuition, and fresh understanding. You can if you think you can, because all the ideas you need to handle any problem are available to you. Cool reactive thinking will open the line of communication. A great combination is sinking in prayer. The main principle is, don't react emotionally—think, think, and think. My motto is: the chief duty of a human being is to master life. You can if you think you can: engrave those seven words deeply in your consciousness. They are packed with power and truth. Self-trust is the first secret of success. There is no life with abandonment. Give all you got and life will give all it has to you. Practice creates this anticipation, the power of positive expectation. Have confidence that you can draw the best, not the worst, to yourself. Be sure to image correctly; we tend to be as we see ourselves. See yourself confidently. Never let any mistake overwhelm you or you stop believing in yourself. Learn from it, let it go, and go on.

# Mindfulness Meditation and Healing

Mindfulness is a state in which the mind is solely focused on what is happening. It is focusing on one thing and not allowing the mind to wander.

When this is done, a deep calm pervades both body and mind. It is a state of mind that needs to be experienced to be understood. Meditation is a way of doing it. Mindfulness can be applied to everything that we do: speeding, driving, doing the dishes, working, and playing. There are endless ways meditate.

The meditator focuses on a certain item—chant, light, word, or object. It results in relaxation and even a state of rapture. Pain may go away, pathological thinking may change, and it may be motivating. Visualizing a change may eliminate a bad habit. Mindfulness is stripping the baggage from the main thing we're dealing with in that moment. No past, no future, no worry or anxiety. True reductionist reasoning; the bare facts. You're concentrating to strip off the wall of illusions that block living in reality. It strips the baggage-accompanying pain, or bad habits, the baggage that causes us to smoke, be fearful, and develop toxic habits.

Mindfulness can be liberating. The breath is generally used as a method of connecting the mind and the body, and is the object of our concentration. Life is a catastrophe, let's face it. In the end it's always a tragedy. Life is filled with constant change; nothing lasts forever. So to constantly act like we are living in a continuous catastrophe is a mistake. We need to learn to live in the moment. Practicing mindfulness and meditation is very helpful. It's the nature of the universe that nothing stays the same. We're too judgmental. Stop judging everything; it's stressful. Everything is not just good, bad, or neutral. They blend into each other, as in the Tao, the Chinese way of thinking. The essence of life is suffering says the Buddhist. Happiness and peace are really the prime issues in human existence. This is what we are seeking, but we cover it up with issues. You can learn to step outside this cycle of wants and desires.

Meditation is intended to purify the mind. It can change the thought process of what we call psychic irritations: greed, hatred, jealousy. Meditation brings the mind to a state of tranquility, awareness, concentration, and insight. Meditation is a great teacher. It's like cultivating a new land. Mindfulness meditation brings together certain attitudes that are essential. We are heading for the bottom line, the truth for the moment. Don't expect anything. In meditational mindfulness awareness, seek to see reality exactly as it is. Feel through the pain, without its baggage. A suspension of all preconceived ideas. No judgment. Let go, accept anything that arises. No hopelessness, no obsession, and above all, no judgment. Question everything except reality. View all problems as challenges. Don't dwell on or obsess about anything.

Start mindful meditation by focusing on your breathing. Pay attention to every aspect of breathing in your practice of mindfulness. You want to practice mindfulness and calm the mind by developing insight and wisdom to realign the truth as it is. You want to know the work of the mind as it really is. You want to get rid of all psychic irritations and annoyances and make your life truly peaceful and happy. Your mind cannot be purified without seeing things as they really are. We should not confuse them with mental formations for body sensations in complexities of the mind. We need to separate the mind and body feelings. When we mindfully watch both body and mind, we can see how many wonderful things they do together.

Mindful practice is the practice of being 100 percent truthful with ourselves. If we are mindful we will be diligent, so we need to look into our own mind. We will be thankful if someone points out our faults. Before we try to surmount our defects, we should know what they are.

Even when we are suffering, we can pretend we are not, or we will not get better. If we are blind to all faults someone needs to point them out to us. If we becomes unmindful to our faults, we will not become better. We should speak mindfully and live mindfully. When we are listening and talking mindfulness, our minds are free from greed, selfishness, hatred, and delusion. Mindfulness is the English translation of the Pali word *sati*. It is an activity, introduced by the Buddha twenty-five centuries ago; a set of mental activity, specifically a sphere of uninterrupted mindfulness. We have developed the habit of squandering and decorating our thoughts with baggage, causing a great deal of stress. Using proper techniques prolongs mindfulness; you find this experience is profound, in that it changes your entire view of the universe. The state of mindfulness can be learned; however, it takes regular practice.

Mindfulness is mirror thought. It reflects only what is presently happening, in exactly the way it is happening. There are no biases. Mindfulness is nonjudgmental observation. It is the ability of the mind to observe without criticism. With this ability, one sees things without condemnation or judgment. One does not decide and does not judge. Mindfulness is an impartial watchfulness. It takes no sides. Mindfulness does not get infatuated with good mental states; it does not try to sidestep the bad mental states. We can use it to break every sort of bad habit we may have or problem that is plaguing us. Mindfulness does not play favorites. Mindfulness is not conceptual awareness. It is bare attention, not thinking. It does not get involved with thoughts or concepts. It does not get hung up on ideas or opinions or memories. Mindfulness registers experiences but does not compare them. Mindfulness is present-moment awareness. Mindfulness is non-egotistic awareness. One just sits back and watches the show. Mindfulness is the observance of the basic nature of each passing phenomena. It works like an electron microscope. Mindfulness sees the transitory and passing nature of everything that is observed.

Apply your attention to the proper object at the proper time and exert precisely the amount of energy needed to do that job. When this energy is properly applied, meditative states conceal a state of calm alertness. There's no greed, lust, or laziness. Be prepared in the mind. Therein lies a mechanism that accepts what the mind experiences that is beautiful and pleasant, and rejects the experiences that are perceived as ugly and painful. This mechanism gives rise to the states of mind that we are training ourselves to avoid.

Mindfulness is attention to present-moment reality and therefore directly the opposite of the day's state of mind that characterizes impediments. Fully developed mindfulness is a state of total nonattachment and utter absence of clinging to anything in the world. It sees things deeply, down below the level of concepts and opinions. The result is a mind that remains unstained and invulnerable, completely undisturbed by the ups and downs of life. The point is that we can use mindfulness to bring happiness, stop toxic habits, develop good health habits, and have a happy, long life with a sound mind.

## Your Own Mind-Body Healer

Having a talk or listening to an imaginary inner advisor may be one of the most powerful techniques for helping you understand the relationship between your thoughts, feelings, actions, and health. There is a doctor living within all of us. Dr. Herb Benson would say, "Let's take advantage of our inner voice." We may have more knowledge in our mind-body than we are aware of. An inner advisor can connect our right and left hemispheres and teach us to learn our minds language, the nonverbal language of symbolism and imagery. Only through a process of self-discovery can you learn to communicate with the deeper parts of yourself to cry out for change. Yet, verbal thoughts are a foreign tongue to your unconscious mind, which communicates through imagery and symbolism. An inner advisor can help you do that. Some use an animation, like a chipmunk, a cat, or a dog. I use one of the primates, an orangutan I have named Einstein. I talk to him regularly when I need advice. Our unconscious mind has more wisdom in it than our conscious mind. Your non-dominant right hemisphere knows precisely what to do when presented with various images and visualizations. When you imagine biting into a lemon slice, for example, what action did it take? It activated the autonomic nervous system center, which is responsible for producing saliva, didn't it?

Bringing things into the realm of the cancer experience, think for a moment of how you envision the problem. You may picture yourself as a helpless, hopeless victim of an incurable disease. We need to change that perception. Your body and immune system know what to do. Remember that there is a doctor living within you. Do not picture yourself as a helpless, hopeless victim of an incurable illness. Do not prepare your right hemisphere with helplessness. Prepare your imagination and visualization by mobilizing the immune and inflammatory defenses that might facilitate healing. The right hemisphere of your brain also picks up cues that you interpret. What you believe will occur. If you have pessimistic thoughts, that makes them come true. Don't let a health-care provider nocebo your health. Don't let "You have only six months to live" get a foothold in your way of thinking. A single picture can be more potent than a dictionary of words. Our brain has tremendous powers of visualization and imagery. You speak to your unconscious mind with images. Take an inner advisor, someone or something you're comfortable with, man or animal or God—your choice. Learn how to contact your inner advisor, and imagine a living creature inhabiting your unconscious mind. This technique—perhaps the most fascinating form of guided imagery—allows you to communicate actively with the nondominant part of your brain, and in turn reach a more complete understanding of the cancer experience. Dr. Bressler in his famous pain book describes a patient who used a hummingbird as an advisor. The right hemisphere of your brain is a vast storehouse of information that can be tremendously useful in healing and curing cancer. The inner advisor can help us change the unconscious belief systems that interfere with our healing. Once you've learned to make conscious contact with your right hemisphere, it's a skill you should never allow to deteriorate. It takes a lot of open-mindedness on your part initially, but you will reap the rewards using guided imagery. An advisor is just a way of talking to ourselves, which is hardly a new concept. Interestingly, children have and use very vivid imagination and it's much easier for them. They naturally communicate with that part of themselves and they constantly create imaginary playmates. Many patients create advisors like Rocky the dog, Merida Tiger, Bambi the deer, Charlie the white rat, Rudy and the orangutan, God, angels, and all sorts of religious symbols. Who you pick is up to you, because it is actually you. As a prerequisite for finding your advisor, it is important to remove yourself from the intrusions of day-to-day life and find a favorite place in your mind's eye— certain room, a place of healing. Perhaps you would like to record your conversation on a CD and play it back to yourself while you're in the car.

When the process begins, take a moment to get comfortable and relaxed. Sit upright in a comfortable chair, feet flat on the floor. Make sure you won't be interrupted for a few minutes. Take the telephone off the hook if necessary. Take a few slow, deep abdominal breaths, and pay attention to your breath as you inhale and exhale. In essence, you are meditating. Breathe in the good, exhale the bad. If you can't quiet your mind, use a mantra; keep repeating the same word and you will relax. Remember your breathing, slow and deep. Paying attention to your breathing will bring you into a state of relaxation, and give you the ability to start your conversation with your advisor. As you allow your body to enjoy this nice state of deep, peaceful relaxation, think of a favorite place (real or imaginary) that's outdoors—beautiful, peaceful, serene, secure, and magical—a special place that you can meet your advisor. As you send serenity all around you, listen to the sounds of nature. As the insects lazily go about their day's work, and the gentle breeze softly begins to touch your face, take a deep breath of the clean, fresh air around you, and enjoy the moment as you exhale. Now that you have found your favorite place, it's time to locate your advisor. There is no better place to seek out your advisor than the calm, peaceful, personal place you've just discovered. Now take the signaled breath, a special message that says you're ready to enter a state of deep relaxation. Breathe in deeply through your nose and exhale through your mouth. Remember your breathing, slow and deep. As you concentrate your attention on your breathing, imagine a ball of pure energy or white light entering your lower abdomen. It rises up to the front of your body, and as you exhale, it moves down your spine, down your legs, into the ground. Each time you inhale and exhale, you may be surprised to find yourself twice as relaxed as you were a moment before, twice as peaceful. With each breath, every cell of your body becomes relaxed. All the tension, tightness, pain, or discomfort drains down your spine. Although your advisor knows everything about you—since your advisor is just a reflection of the inner life—tell your advisor what you are trying to accomplish, ask for his advice, and then do what he recommends that you do. In other words, we communicate, we believe, and we make it happen. The doctor living inside you who controls your immunity can increase your lifespan and your chances of a spontaneous healing.

The advisor is our inner wisdom and experience. He is a friendly guide for our unconscious stores of knowledge. Gut feelings and the voice within us are examples of our unconscious thoughts. Imaging or visualizing an advisor makes the process more acceptable and accessible. An inner advisor can be the bridge between the conscious and unconscious mind. Many cultures use rituals that include music, chanting, and dancing to invoke a vision to guide them. Catholic children are taught to have a guardian angel to help and advise them.

Whatever you believe—that your advisor is a spirit, a guardian angel, a messenger from God, or a command between the left and right sides of the brain—it does not matter. It can help you. I speak to my advisor daily; he rides around with me in the passenger seat of my car most of the day, between hospitals and when I'm coming and going. The advisor can act as a source of inner calm and comfort, a companion, and you may feel a sense of peace. Talk to your advisor when you get up and when you go to bed. It'll make you feel better. Remember, I named my advisor Einstein. When I have a tough operation or stressful day, I speak to him and ask his advice and encouragement. It's a step to a better day. If things go particularly well I thank him. Working with an advisor can result in a healing or the relief of symptoms, and may be a cure. We all have an advisor living within us. There is a doctor inside us, take advantage of it. As I've already said, the advisor can be a spirit, your God, a cartoon figure, or an animal—it doesn't really matter. As the real Einstein said, "Imagination is more important than knowledge."

## Healing the Mind with Art

Emotions have a direct impact on your body. Every one of your one hundred billion brain cells and trillions of nerve transmitters speak to your body, and every one of your seventy billion body cells speak in turn to your brain. Mind-body, body-mind. Visualization is a great way to increase our communicating system between the body and the mind, and the mind and the body. It takes advantage of a huge ability to visualize an image to communicate with our unconscious mind and to connect the right and left sides of the brain. There is a doctor living in our unconscious and we need to put him to work. Visualization is a great medium because it uses images of the imaginative right hemisphere and connects it to the doing part of our brain, the left hemisphere, which gets the job done.

As this illustration demonstrates, it releases the eagle within you. Avoid blame; it will make you feel powerless. The flip side of blame is responsibility. Don't blame yourself for eating the wrong food or smoking most of your life; take full responsibility for it and try to do something about it. No one consciously picks his or her disease, nor does he or she consciously create it. Dr. Deepak Chopra says, in his book *Quantum Healing*, that doctors can cut out cancer or treat it with chemo, but it will return if the emotions and conditions that caused the cancer are not dealt with by the patient.

With art you can learn to transfer your emotions onto the canvas and deal with them. Whether they are positive or negative, a visual representation of them will help you create a change. You can draw positive and negative images, and convert one to the other. Constructing positive images that you paint can stimulate the process and awaken the immune system within you to lead to the healing. To heal your body, you must heal your mind first. There are three main steps in healing with art, according to Barbara Gannon, and I quote her work liberally. You can use the acronym ART.

1. **A**ccess the images of your stress-producing feelings and emotions by visualizing them as inner images.
2. **R**elease these emotions and feelings by expressing the images that represent them through art.
3. **T**ransform the images of your negative thoughts and painful emotions into positive and empowering images.

# Materials

You may want to put a variety of art materials out in front of you before you begin, and once you have done this visualization, you can then allow your emotions to guide you in selecting an appropriate medium of art. If you're feeling more like squeezing, pounding, or pushing your emotions out of your body, try some clay. As you look at the art you've just created that expresses the stress-producing emotions you have been holding in a particular part of your body, what does this tell you about these emotions? How do you feel when you look at this artwork? What does your choice of colors tell you about the emotion or emotions being expressed in your artwork? I would visualize art on a canvas; you're fighting the cancer with whatever weapons you decide to choose. If you see it in the mind, it is much more likely to happen. Look at the weapons destroying your cancer cells every day in your imagination as well as on the canvas. Transformation is the third step in dealing with art. To transform means to change. You're changing the way you react to painful emotion. Also, you are producing the healing effect. Look at the image as expressed in a drawing or painting of stress-producing emotions or your army, navy, and air force fighting the cancer daily. The ability to visualize and your imaging ability are huge, and art is a great way to put these to work in order to double your lifespan and increase the spontaneous cure rate.

You need to connect with the inner voice of your spirit, passing through art the imagistic messages of your heart. By turning to your body's energy system, you will learn how to open the connection between your soul and universal spirit energy. This connection will allow you to communicate directly with your soul. Using art to express its messages, you can discover your divine purpose on this planet, and despite all that has happened in your life, good and bad, you will be in harmony with this purpose. You will learn unconditional love and forgiveness, which brings the process of healing and transformation of body, mind, and spirit full circle.

## Patient Survival Stories

Cancer is a word in my vocabulary that has a different meaning to me now because I am a survivor, with so much to share with anyone who is facing the same journey. I feel it to be my mission to help newly diagnosed cancer patients understand the complex emotions they will experience, and give them the hope they need to channel themselves in the right direction—the direction forward, toward a healthy post-cancer state where they, too, are a survivor.

All people have a fear that they will one day become ill with a fatal disease that takes over and leaves them weak and vulnerable, without hope. The first sign that something could be wrong—the discovery of a lump in the breast, neck, or armpit—is sometimes appreciated in the subconscious as an affirmation that it was there before, or maybe something they just did not notice. The night sweats are just because we could be starting menopause. Fatigue is rather common these days because no one gets enough sleep. This is a state of denial. Denial is a safety zone where we temporarily stop in to seek shelter when a storm is eminent. We want to believe everything is really normal. And this is, alas, a bad dream which we will wake up from, and it will be morning with the sun shining.

The diagnosis of cancer is a rough one to get over. It is like the day Kennedy was assassinated, or September 11, for we will never forget that day; the weather, the people involved, or exactly how we were told. Let us hope the messenger was compassionate. This begins the long journey. Disbelief is the word commonly used to describe this take-your-breath-away moment. This is the turning point where suddenly we discover what it is like to be told our life could be over. Dramatic, for we are now a statistic and officially sick. What was once a glimmer of hope is now an overwhelming challenge to our mental state. This is a good time for us to lose it and cry a lot, sob profusely, and go through the "Why me? I take good care of myself!" speech. Thank goodness for friends and family who will talk us down off the ledge. Here starts the healing process, where love and compassion give us the strength to go on and face what is ahead with the energy we receive from acts of kindness. Throughout the duration of the illness we are constantly regenerated with the positive flow of energy when we are around the people who make this stressful time tolerable. Whether they be the medical caregivers, family, friends, neighbors, or even the mailman, when they ask, "How are you doing today?" they really mean what they say. Cancer can bring out the best in people. Love is a healing mechanism. Love is an energy that fills a room. Love releases endorphins that feel like the rush we get from a steroid high, only safer and with long-lasting aftereffects.

Looking back, a frequently asked question was, "Do you have friends or family?" We all need to be surrounded by a support group at this time. Desperation is a lonely and hollow emotion, twice as difficult without someone holding our hand. Remembering back, I will never forget my sister reaching over and rubbing my back as I waited for the first chemotherapy to begin. It still brings me to tears. That moment of love and tenderness gave me the strength and courage to hold my breath and jump in the deep end and begin the treatment that would save my life. The power of the human touch is so awesome. We all respond to touch. It can arouse us, give us goose bumps, tickle, even at times repulse. A pat on the back is a commonly used phrase describing affirmation. A comforting massage relaxes us and stimulates circulation, even lymphatic response. Massage gives our mind a sense of well-being and serenity. Critically ill babies benefit from a mother's touch. The power of touch during cancer is very important. I remember my oncologist affectionately rubbing the top of my bald head. This small gesture was so important because I really knew that he cared about me. This speaks volumes, because my oncologist was my hero. After accepting the fact that I did indeed have cancer, I then asked myself what I was going to do about it. Like everything else in my life, I decided that cancer did not own me, and no way would I cower again. I did not want to lose, because I am a competitive and motivated personality. My challenge was to claim ownership and take control. Cancer was not going to run my life. When my hair started to fall out I recoiled in terror, but after a few days of that, it was time to shave it off and get over it. Here, the decision was made by me to be proactive and beat cancer with a checkmate strategy. I was going to outwit it with my get-it-done-and-over-with mentality. My thoughts were, *It will grow back. It is only hair.* I discovered a new, emancipated me. The question was then answered. This was the real me. I am not my hair. I am not my clothes or my career. I am a soul, my mother's daughter, a sister, a friend, and I am loved. I did not want to die and cancer would not define me. Wigs were not an option. Too hot for me, and it was what it was at the time. I had no shame. Why cover up or disguise my cancer? Everyone that knows me was aware of the fact. Letting go of the hair was easier for me because my clients have been through it, so I knew the inevitable would happen and I accepted the challenge. Staying one step ahead, I went into my control-freak mode, decided that getting well was my ultimate goal, and started to envision myself well again, fast-forwarding myself six months into the future. The chemotherapy would be over, and as my hair returned, so would my health.

During my six months of chemotherapy, I walked into a new world of hospitals and waiting rooms filled with people in treatment, all wearing the same hairstyle. At first, I was disturbed by the sight of hairless women in mass quantities until I realized we all were members of the same unique sorority of sorts. Once strangers, we knew one another without talking. Our energy in the room was invigorating, for we had all assembled together for the same common purpose. We must move toward a better state of wellness. The energy in the room was generated by all the beautiful people who had come in support of their loved one. My sisters, who always came with me in support, would acknowledge other caregivers in the room as if they were soldiers in the same army. It was very interesting to watch the people interact within the groups: husbands supporting wives, wives supporting husbands, sister supporting sister, daughter supporting mother, mother supporting daughter, friend supporting friend. We all shared the common bond of love that would fuel the fire of hope.

During this time, when my body was weakened by the side effects of treatment, I would retreat to my inner soul. The mind is a powerful thing during this period. There is a lot of time to think and reflect when you are waiting for the drugs to slowly drip into your veins. What else is there to do as you lie in a PET scan for forty-five minutes? Waiting rooms are not just for waiting. I was very introspective at this time, for my once hectic life had come to a temporary pause. There was a reason for me to be here, only to live in the now and get my life back together. I would look toward the future, making plans for everything I needed to finish before life got away from me. It was time for the bucket list. I really must get to Italy, but first I need to apologize to a few people, take more time off work, spend more time with the people I love, and maybe not worry so much about my retirement IRA. Things are not as important as relationships now; money cannot buy health; love does conquer all. The moral support from family and friends plays a significant part in cancer treatment. It is critical to maintain a positive attitude and, most importantly, remain in a mental state of projection into a healthy body once again. I would always mentally fast-forward past the chemotherapy into remission. I still am looking forward to year five cancer free, when I can own the word *remission* as the new word of choice in my life. At that point, I can honestly say that I am in remission and leave the word *cancer* at rest-

By Carol Lynn

Sarah is just one of the many faces of cancer in my circle of friends. I have known her from a distance for many years, and when she was diagnosed with lung cancer, I extended my hand to help her transition through the hair loss. I did not know Sarah well because she suffered from clinical depression and never really left the comfort zone of her home after her son's suicide. I only knew her from the conversations with her husband, a client of mine for many years. He always spoke to me out of concern, for the Sarah he once knew seemed to be missing, and her existence was now limited to the confines of her bedroom, with an occasional visit downstairs. I would often wonder when she would snap out of it, but this went on for years.

When she was diagnosed, I thought she would plummet into deeper despair, and I was wrong. Her husband's relentless love and devotion sustains her, and her family and friends hold her in a safe place as they wrap her in love and support. The task of cutting falling locks is always difficult, yet inevitable. Usually the cancer patient is hesitant to let go of her identity as the limp locks trickle to the floor, and reminisces about the past, when things seemed carefree. A better time before cancer dimmed the lights. Sarah was different because she was going from bad to worse. I expected to see an emotional Sarah. I was happy to see a strong and composed Sarah, with high hopes for a recovery and second chance in life. It often seems to be the case that we don't know what we've got until it's gone. During the haircut, I was privileged to share her thoughts about her destiny. How inspirational for me, for I was reminded once again how beautiful and too short life is, and that I, too, was spared after my own battle with cancer.

In her own words: "For once, after years of hell grieving for my son, I want to live now. For the first time I REALLY feel the love from the people who are important to me, and I do not want to leave them. I want to beat this and start my life over again." This is very common with cancer patients. I felt the same way, and have my own "bucket list." It has been a year since Sarah was diagnosed, and she has seen better days health-wise, and hope sustains her when she stumbles through the endless stays at chemo and radiation. Her journey has been long and tedious, and recently she faced another challenge with dementia as a result of radiation to the brain. As you well know, the radiation was a precautionary measure. I was again commissioned to color and cut her new hair, which was very much needed to boost her morale. Again, I did not know what to expect. She was in rehab at a nursing home. How depressing. Her cancer was back again, and her husband chose not to tell her. I agreed this was a good decision. It was difficult for me to go back to the same nursing home that had swallowed my father up ten years earlier. I remembered all the times I entered the doors of that same hall to find a stranger of the dad I once knew, hoping he would recognize me as his daughter. He never did, but he always asked me for the keys to his car so he could go home. Dad eventually went home to heaven.

When entering the same door I had entered years ago, it was hard, for I felt a sense of despair due to the memories of my past visits haunting me. Little did I know my despair would soon turn the corner as I entered her room. Sitting in a wheelchair I saw a somewhat familiar face of hope as Sarah smiled and welcomed me into her world. Her husband stood beside her with a boyish grin, yet looked somewhat sad, knowing the secret he was keeping from her. My heart was heavy, for standing on her other side was her grandson, Evan, the son of her deceased son who had taken his own life. Suicide always leaves so many emotional scars for the surviving family. How ironic that the emotional scars left behind by his death had finally been healed with cancer. I will never forget rinsing Sarah's hair as her husband playfully grabbed her hand. That simple sign of affection warmed my heart as I remembered the same signs of love during my own cancer treatment. Those simple things speak volumes to cancer patients. Even a smile from the doctor can change their day. Going into the much-anticipated haircut, Sarah talked about her battle with cancer and how much she appreciated the people around her who have made her well with their love. She commented with joy that she almost died, and how happy she was to be spared and have a second chance. That second chance seems to be key in recovering from cancer. As I cut her hair, I could see she was filled with hope, and there was no sign of dementia. Sarah seemed emotionally committed to getting back home. I commented on the pictures her husband had hung on the walls and all the beautiful flowers. Her husband is a saint! He had enlarged a picture of Sarah to poster size. The picture was from twenty years ago, when they first met. She was holding a single rose and smiling. I am sure the rose was from John, her husband, for her smile was a mile wide. He made the comment that he wanted the nursing staff to know Sarah for the person she was. She certainly looked more like the old Sarah after I covered her gray locks and gave her a new style. That chemo cut is never very flattering. Sarah is now home and wakes John in the night with her rattling, disturbing, and relentless cough. She thinks she has a cold. She looks forward to the morning because the cough gets worse when she lies down.

## Patient Survival Stories

There's nothing like hearing stories from patients who practice mind-body techniques, as well as from their doctors who have used them. The medical community in general does not accept mind-body techniques to heal cancer. There are now, though, many famous cancer centers where it is part of every case. I do not exclusively treat cancer, but see some patients with it every week. A significant amount of cancer goes to the brain and spine and that is what I treat. I try to teach almost every cancer patient I have personal contact with about the effect of their mind on the cancer.

In my experience this gives them hope. I put some smiles on their faces and actually have improved the outcome in a significant number of the patients, including a few spontaneous cures. At the moment I'm treating a metastatic lung cancer to the spine. When I initially saw her, she looked so depressed, but I gave her Dr. Carl Simonton's book to read and I notice she is smiling more and a lot more hopeful. Most of the radiation techs and medical oncologists have admitted to me that they do not know a great deal about the connection of the mind and cancer. It is not part of their medical training.

Dr. Carl Simonton's first patient is a fascinating story. I mean the first patient on which he tried his developing theories about the mind-body connection and healing with cancer.

He was a sixty-one-year-old man who, in 1971, came to the medical school with a form of throat cancer and a grave prognosis. He was very weak and was not expected to live very long. He weighed ninety-eight pounds, could barely swallow his own saliva, and had difficulty breathing. A less than 5 percent chance of living five years. Doctors even considered not treating him. Dr. Carl taught the patient to help himself with relaxation techniques, meditation techniques, visualization, and imaging based on his research. The patient did that five to fifteen minutes, three times a day. Dr. Carl asked him to picture his treatment, radiation therapy, as consisting of millions of tiny bullets of energy that would hit his cells, both normal and cancerous, that got in the path of the X-ray beam, because the cancer cells when weakened would not be able to repair themselves, and the normal cells would return to health. Dr. Carl then asked the patient to form a mental picture of his healing white cells coming in, swarming over the cancer cells, picking up and carrying off the dead and dying cells, flushing them out of his body through the liver and kidneys. In his mind's eye, he would visualize the cancer decreasing in size and his breathing returned to normal. The radiation treatments worked exceptionally well; almost no skin change, no hair lost, and halfway through the treatments the patient was able to eat and gain weight. The cancer essentially disappeared. Interestingly enough, the patient used imaging techniques to get rid of his arthritis and also cured his impotency with that technique.

You can see why Dr. Carl became excited and motivated to publish this and to use this method on his patients. Another two patients of Dr. Carl's had similar illnesses. They both had lung cancer spread to the brain. The first patient received a diagnosis and resigned from life. He quit his job, settled in front of the TV set, staring blankly hour after hour at the clock so that he would take his pain medication on time. No one could get him interested in anything. He did not respond to radiation or chemotherapy and was dead in three months.

Patient number two also had lung cancer that had spread to the brain, and the prognosis was the same. Patient number two responded totally different. He reviewed his priorities in life. He had been a salesman and frankly had not stopped to look at the trees in all that time. He continued to work part-time and took some time off. He practiced imaging and visualization techniques daily and participated in group therapy. He lived many years, which is not usually expected with metastatic lung cancer. I have had numerous patients with lung cancer that spread to the brain. I have found whenever the patients get the idea that I really care about them, that I love them—give them CDs to listen to, DVDs to watch, and some books to read about the mind and cancer—they live a lot longer and the spontaneous cure rate goes up.

Here is another great story from Dr. Carl. Edie, a forty-year-old woman, came to the hospital with advanced cancer of the kidney. She had been widowed during the preceding year, but continued to live and work on the ranch left to her by her husband. An exploratory operation revealed that she had cancer that had spread outside the kidney, and it would be impossible to remove it surgically. She was treated with minimal doses of radiation, but there was little expectation for improvement. Remember, death of a spouse results in an increased rate of cancer. She was sent home to the ranch, after being given only a few months to live. Once home, she fell in love with one of the men working on the ranch and they were soon married. Despite the prognosis of imminent death, she showed no further signs of the illness for five years. Then, her second husband left her after running through her money. Within a few weeks she had a major recurrence of cancer and died shortly thereafter. It would seem that her remarriage played a significant role in her apparent recovery, and that being deserted precipitated the recurrence of the disease and her death.

Dr. Khalsa speaks about a patient who thought she had brought lung cancer upon herself and was afraid she would cause it to recur or to spread. That's the reason she went to see Dr. Khalsa He related that as she approached seventy and mandatory retirement age, as well as being an elementary school teacher, students seemed to annoy her more and her work became unpleasant. Unmarried, she shared her apartment with another older woman, whom she also found increasingly annoying. Her whole world seemed to be deteriorating. She noticed that she began smoking more, and that as she inhaled the smoke, she was thinking it wouldn't be long until she would be dead. For several months, she continued to smoke and became more and more depressed. She developed an increasingly severe cough that eventually produced some blood.

Then she was found to have lung cancer and underwent surgery. After the operation, her depression recurred, and as a result she became apprehensive about the possibility of recurring disease, which she so strongly believed she had participated in developing in the first place. When she voiced this to her surgeon, he remembered Dr. Carl's lecture and referred her for consultation. This patient was the first one to tell Dr. Carl she had made herself ill, and could relate the actual thought process she had experienced. Having previously undergone some psychotherapy, she was aware of her thoughts and feelings. She required very little help in overcoming her fear and depression.

Dr. Carl also mentions that many of the patients who develop conflicts with their spouses, like an affair or death, are much more likely to develop cancer. Several male patients who developed conflicts centering on their business were found to have higher cancer rates. He talks about a patient named Rod who received his cancer diagnosis within a year after his business began to deteriorate. Dr. Carl taught him how to deal with these problems more directly and the healing began. Another frequent life pattern found in cancer patients is that of a woman who had invested all her emotional and much of her physical energy into her family. She was the chauffeur, cook, nursemaid, and counselor to her four children, including ballet classes, music lessons, football games, slumber parties, and PTA meetings. When it was all over, she developed cancer. The husband had been a successful executive with a major corporation who had to travel a great deal; responsibility for the children fell almost entirely on her. When it was all over, cancer was the rewarding purpose!

Dr. Carl speaks about a patient named Janet, who was diagnosed with breast cancer that had spread to her abdominal cavity. She began using visual imagery when she entered therapy. Despite this serious prognosis, she had a remarkably good response and was able to return to work and resume her normal activities for two and a half years. Janet then began to experience some emotional upsets, and after several months of unusual stress the disease flared up again. During an imaging session shortly thereafter, she visualized the image of her white blood cells and asked them to work overtime in a specific effort to regain control of her tumor. They replied that they would not work alone, that she would have to work with them. They indicated that if she were to regain her health, it was important that she get in touch with the emotional reasons why her disease was recurring and do something about them, in addition to practicing imaging three times a day. Then they reassured her that they would continue to work diligently to cure her cancer and would reproduce so there would be a continuous source of new white blood cells to fight her disease. As a result of this dialogue, she returned to the Simonton Center for a follow-up therapy session as she began to uncover and deal with the recent difficulties. During the session, the tumor began to diminish and she returned home, again on the road to recovery.

Francis is another patient who reported engaging in an internal dialogue with the visual imagery. Frances came to the Simonton Center after being diagnosed with a recurrence of lymphoma, a cancer that affects the lymphatic system. As part of imagery, she imagined her cancer being destroyed by chemotherapy and the white blood cells. Then she would imagine her bone marrow remaining healthy and producing white blood cells to combat the cancer. Francis is a poet and kept a journal for ideas, intuitions, and dreams.

Dr. Bernie S. Siegel tells an amazing story about his patient Gladys. She had a chronic intestinal inflammation for some fifty years, and learned to manipulate her whole family. He met her after she developed cancer. She had a family member waiting on her twenty-four hours a day. Even when they hired a nurse to take care of her, Gladys would awaken the family and let the nurse sleep. Over and over she developed severe pains at home, which mysteriously disappeared each time she was admitted to the hospital. Nearly every weekend she would have those who were not at home during the week in the emergency room with her to help evaluate her returning chest pains. Thus, those who worked during the week got their share. When Dr. Siegel was counseling her, she would get someone to hand her a glass of water or a tissue, even when what she wanted was only inches away. Dr. Siegel gave her *The Will to Live*, the famous book by Dr. Arnold Hutschnecker. The next morning when he returned on his rounds, she said she had forgotten the book. The message was clear: "Please don't try to teach me to give up my illness, because it's the only way I can relate to people." Learning to love was frightening. He kept trying to reach Gladys, and she said he was the only doctor who ever gave her hope. Truthfully, he thought he was the only one who continued to care for her without being worn-out by the constant manipulation, which included side effects of every medication he recommended. He learned to let her do much of the talking, and recommend things that fit her belief system. Then he would always get the credit and be called a wonderful doctor. Finally, during one of her phone calls, he told her he had a new drug that would cure her cancer. He asked her to come to the office, since it had to be given by injection. He did this after explaining his plan to the family and asked them to watch Gladys reaction. He was trying to save them from being the victims of her illness. She never did make it to the office and canceled the majority of her appointments.

It's important to realize that we can't force others to change; we can only help them to change themselves. This is a point I finally learned after many years of dealing with patients. It is generally said among those in the medical community that 70 percent of the patients don't wish to participate in their health care. I don't accept that. Health-care providers need to be motivators, and in my experience there are ways to do it. Dr. Siegel's point is not to judge the patient's motives, but to bring him or her out in the open and perhaps he or she will change. When you think about it, our insurance system rewards you when you take a sick day, not a health day. When trying to cure yourself of cancer, or at least participate in it, pessimism is a luxury you can't afford.

Dr. Bernie Siegel speaks about taking three ECaPs—exceptional cancer patients, willing to participate in their health care—onto the *Phil Donahue* TV show to tell their stories. One of those three patients met a former boyfriend in Chicago, stayed, and married him. She chose not to have radiation therapy for breast cancer. She's alive and well today, and Dr. Siegel felt that her remarriage and redirection of her life helped save her. The second, who had had cancer twice, also is free of disease. Mind you, these are patients who participated in relaxation therapy, cognitive therapy, imaging, and visualization. The third patient, named Melanie, later died—but not of cancer; rather, from a treatment complication, an infection after a bone marrow transplant. Her story began during a divorce, when her husband asked her how she was doing. She said, "I'm having a very difficult time," and he said, "Oh, you look terrific." She thought, *I'll never share anything with him again.* She held her feelings inside and developed leukemia. She made a very significant change in lifestyle thereafter. Many times, when a physician thought she would not survive, she did. This happened so often that later on, when it really looked as though she wouldn't make it and physicians reinforced her beliefs that they expected her to recover, she did once more. She got to the point where she literally ran out of chemotherapy options, because she had so many remissions. Finally, she underwent a bone marrow transplant, which was unusual considering her age. Dr. Siegel sent a letter to the hospital, explaining what an exceptional patient she was. They accepted her and learned from her that age alone is not a significant issue, but rather your will to live and survival characteristics. She gave them all a lesson in how to behave as an exceptional cancer patient.

Dr. Siebert found that the survivor personality could be learned, although it can't be taught the way algebra or chemistry is. He conceived of it as a broad process of psychological and neurological maturation, growing up that actually involves remaining a child. It means being childlike and childish. He means playfulness for its own sake, like that of a happy childhood. To lose track of time, external events, and all your worries; often whistling, humming, or talking to yourself absentmindedly; having a child's innocent curiosity and an observant, nonjudgmental style; developing an active imagination, daydreaming, and participating in conversations with yourself.

# Summary

You've been diagnosed with cancer, or someone you know has been; your friend, a relative, maybe your mother or father or brother or sister.

If you've read this book, I hope I've opened your eyes and your mind to follow the mind-body map that I have provided for you to start healing. What do you have to lose? Let's encourage your army, navy, and air force—your immunity—to get to work. Many of the great physicians that I've referenced in this book—including myself, in my forty-two years of experience of treating patients—have seen the power of positive thinking. Dr. Carl Simonton, Dr. Lawrence LeShan, Dr. Bernie Siegel, and many others have proven this, along with scientific studies. How your mind responds to the diagnosis, positively or negatively, will make a huge difference in your longevity and spontaneous cure rate. As Dr. Siegel says, become an exceptional cancer patient. Dr. Norman Vincent Peale spent his life teaching positive thinking. I've read all his books three times and am totally convinced of the positive mind power. He was so convinced of it that he built a psychiatric institute next to his church, which incidentally is still there. He always said, "You can if you think you can."

You need to find a reason for living, a purpose. Set a long-term goal. The Rev. Rick Warren was correct in his famous book *The Purpose Driven Life*. He felt the most healing purpose was helping others.

Convert your mind to a creative one, not a destructive one.

The will to live is inside all of us; wake it up if it's asleep. As Dr. Herb Benson said, "There lives a doctor within all of us."

Get rid of negative thoughts and ignore the nocebo—negative speak—of such statements as "You have only a year to live." No one knows our lifespan for sure, there are exceptions to everything, and I've seen it many times. Most cancers are treatable; be an exceptional cancer patient.

Of course, participate in your standard medical treatment. I encourage you to get multiple opinions. God provides them for you.

You have to find a loving, caring medical provider, a holistic healer. It will make a difference.

Develop a team of great social support. Join group therapy if possible. I hope you have a big family of support, including friends and neighbors.

Your spirituality is critical to your outcome. Speak to your religious leader frequently, and believe in the power of prayer. I pray with my patients frequently.

Consider developing the "healing advisor" concept as described. Human, animal, or God, it doesn't matter; communicate frequently and follow the advice. The concept of developing a healing advisor can be very helpful.

Visualize an image of your immunity force coming in and destroying your cancer, five to fifteen minutes, three times a day, frequently.

Stress control is important. Use Dr. Rudy's twenty prescriptions for stress reduction given in this book or print them off the Web site, www.kachmannmindbody.com.

Sugar is a cancer fuel. I highly recommend eating the nutrient-dense diet as described in my book, *The Secret of the Non Diet*, or read the book *Super Immunity* by Dr. Joel Fuhrman.

Exercise daily—walk, dance, do yoga, tai chi, or chi-gong, and use some light weights.

Love and hopefulness are healing. Hopelessness is destructive. Depression leads to death.

Optimism, positive thinking, spirituality, a great social network, and receiving proper medical treatment can double your lifespan and increase your cure rate. It has been scientifically proven.

Good luck, and I want you to know that I love you, and I thank you for participating in the healing.

# Mind-Body Healing Cancer Mind Map

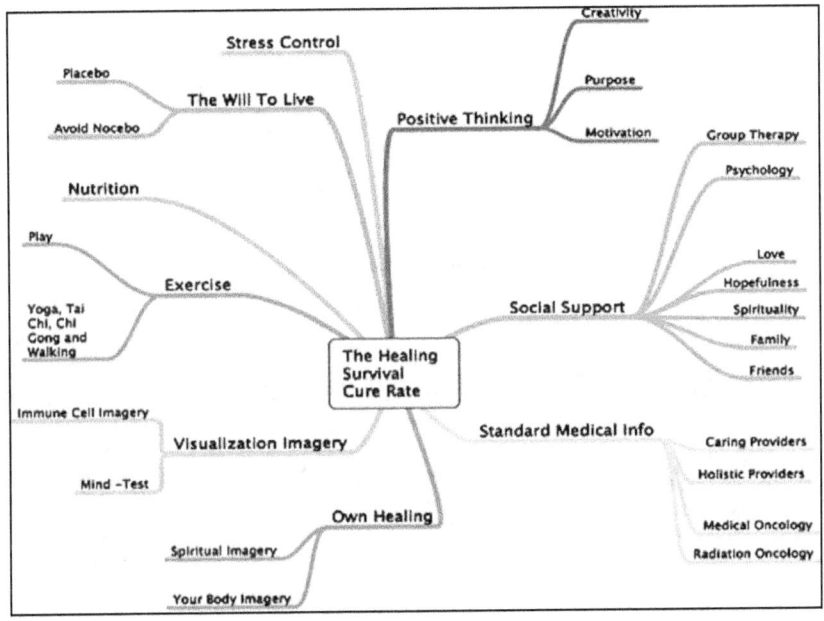

# Dr. Kachmann's Twenty Daily Prescriptions to Reduce Stress

1.  CREATE A SPIRITUAL SAFE PLACE IN YOUR HOME
    a.  Three minutes of abdominal breathing that is calm and focused.

2.  MEDITATE
    a.  Concentrate on your nasal breath.
    b.  Next concentrate on your abdomen going up and down.
    c.  Say or chant a mantra (mind energy) multiple times. For example: Spirit, God, Om, Sat Nam, Let Go, Be Free, I'm Happy, etc.

3.  VISUALIZE AN IMAGE DAILY OF WHAT YOU WANT TO ACHIEVE THAT DAY OR IN THE FUTURE

4.  SAY SOMETHING THANKFUL WHEN YOU GO TO BED EVERY NIGHT AND SAY SOMETHING OPTIMISTIC OR JOYFUL EVERY MORNING

5.  MANAGE YOUR FINANCES WELL BECAUSE THESE ARE ONE OF THE BIGGEST CAUSES OF STRESS
    a.  Get your finances organized.
    b.  Don't panic and remember to breathe.
    c.  Be disciplined and know your debts.
    d.  Make a new plan by thinking your way out of it and seeing a new way of making it.

6.  DON'T FOCUS ON NEGATIVITY
    a.  Avoid TV, radio, and bad news media. Go one a media fast.
    b.  Don't spend the whole night on the computer or watching TV. Give yourself time to transition into sleep—read a book, relax, and let the mind unwind.

c. News media are preoccupied with gloom and doom, crime, world pain, murder, mayhem and perversion. Give it a rest.

7. PRACTICE YOGA, TAI CHI, WALK, DANCE, OR ENJOY EXERCISES THAT BRING ABOUT RELAXATION AND MEDITATION RATHER THAN OVERSTRESSING THE BODY AND MIND

8. EACH DAY SPEND FIFTEEN TO THIRTY MINUTES PRACTICING MEDITATIVE WALKING ("WALKING MEDITATION")
   a. Use your senses to explore the present moment.
   b. Appreciate sounds, appreciate what you see, and appreciate nature.

9. THINK POSITIVELY
   a. Be hardheaded and tough-minded; refuse to let others bring you down.
   b. Don't give up; believe in yourself.
   c. Make a plan to solve the problem.
   d. Write a plan and visualize it daily.

10. LIVE IN THE PRESENT MOMENT, NOT IN THE FUTURE OR THE PAST
    a. Live in the light of the day, not in the storm of yesterday and tsunami of tomorrow.

11. ENJOY MUSIC IN YOUR HOME AND IN YOUR CAR ON THE WAY TO WORK AND BACK
    a. It is the language of God or Spirit.
    b. Music sound is medicine. It is the bridge between spirit and matter.

12. EAT PROPER FOOD
    a. Food is a drug—don't abuse it.

b. Don't use food to manage your psychology because it is not a good stress reducer.

c. Read *The Secret of the Non Diet*. It is about proper food selection.

13. ORGANIZE YOUR TIME
   a. Demand at least fifteen to thirty minutes for yourself daily, no matter what the situation is.

14. TREAT YOURSELF TO A MASSAGE, LET GO OF THE MONKEY MIND
   a. Take a mind shampoo and clean your mind of stress daily. How you think is everything.

15. DON'T SMOKE, USE ILLEGAL DRUGS, OR EXCESSIVE MEDICATIONS
   a. In the long run, they will cause stress.

16. FALL IN LOVE WITH YOURSELF AND APPRECIATE THE LOVE OF THE FAMILY, NO MATTER WHAT THE PROBLEMS ARE

17. BE A HAPPY PERSON
   a. Avoid negative thoughts or statements. No one can solve all the worlds' problems, so don't focus on them.

18. LIVE THE LIFE OF GRATITUDE RATHER THAN A LIFE OF REGRET
   a. You can't change the past.
   b. Say nice things to people all day, like, "You look great," "Have a nice day," or "Thank you again."

19. LET GO OF SELF-JUDGMENT AND SELF-CRITICISM
   a. You are the creation of spirit or God. He does not make mistakes.

20. KNOW WHAT MIND-BODY ILLNESSES OR STRESS-RELATED
ILLNESSES ARE

   a. Stress causes 75 percent of the illnesses that we see a doctor about.
Wellness and stress education is what you need 75 percent of the
time.

   b. Avoid unnecessary tests and procedures.

   c. By understanding what the illnesses are, I have gathered them
together in the mind-body index.

   d. Read *Welcome to Your Mind Body*. It will save you money in
medical care, reduce your stress, and cure your problems with
the proper techniques as recommended above.

# Visit www.kachmannmindbody.com for a list of all Dr. Kachmann's books and DVDs.

**Books:**

*The Call of Life*
*The Fraud of Alzheimer's Disease* (also available on DVD)
*Nocebo: Placebo's Evil Twin* (also available on DVD and CD)
*The Secret of the Non Diet for Adults* (also available on DVD and CD)
*The Secret of the Non Diet for Children* (also available on DVD and CD)
*Kid Scripts: Just What the Doctor Ordered*
*The Psychology of Eating* (also available on DVD and CD)
*Reversing Type 2 Diabetes in 60 Days* (also available on DVD and CD)
*Welcome to Your Mind Body* (also available on DVD and CD)
*Secrets of Motivating Yourself to Wellness* (also available on DVD and CD)
*The Fraud of Chronic Pain*

**DVDs:**

*The Mind and Stress* (also available on CD)
*Living Healthier and Longer* (also available on CD)
*Chinese Medicine* (also available on CD)
*Acute and Chronic Pain* (also available on CD)
*Smoking Cessation* (also available on CD)
*True Vitality* (DVD only)
*Secrets of the Mind and Cancer* (DVD only)

**Now Available:**

Magic 5 of Longevity. This set of five books, handpicked by Dr. Kachmann, will provide you with his proven secrets of everything you need for perfect health and looks.

Magic 5 of Pain Control. This DVD set includes not only holistic treatments for pain reduction but a way to live a stress-free life using mindfulness-based approaches.

**All of these titles, and many more, can be found and purchased online at www.kachmannmindbody.com, shop.kachmannmindbody.com, www.amazon.com and more.**

www.ingramcontent.com/pod-product-compliance
Lightning Source LLC
Chambersburg PA
CBHW071325310526
45789CB00016B/754